KUNDALINI MEDITATION

The path to personal transformation and creativity

KATHRYN McCUSKER

WATKINS PUBLISHING

LONDON

Kundalini Meditation
Kathryn McCusker

Distributed in the USA and Canada by
Sterling Publishing Co., Inc.
387 Park Avenue South
New York, NY 10016-8810

This edition first published in the UK and USA in 2013 by
Watkins Publishing Limited
Sixth Floor
75 Wells Street
London W1T 3QH

A member of Osprey Group

Managing Editor: Sandra Rigby
Senior Editor: Fiona Robertson
Managing Designer: Luana Gobbo
Designer: Peggy Sadler
Picture Research: Emma Copestake
Commissioned Artwork: Paolo d'Altan
Commissioned Photography: Jules Selmes
Make-up Artist: Justine Martin

ISBN: 978-1-78028-530-6

10 9 8 7 6 5 4 3 2 1

Typeset in Joanna MT and Baskerville
Color reproduction by Imagewrite
Printed in Singapore by Imago

For information about custom editions, special sales, premium and corporate purchases, please
contact Sterling Special Sales Department at 800-805-5489 or specialsales@sterlingpub.com.

Publisher's note: The information in this book is not intended as a substitute for
professional medical advice and treatment. If you are pregnant or are suffering from
any medical conditions or health problems, it is recommended that you consult a
medical professional before following any of the advice or practice suggested in this
book. Watkins Publishing Ltd., or any other persons who have been involved in working
on this publication, cannot accept responsibility for any injuries or damage incurred as
a result of following the information, exercises or therapeutic techniques contained in
this book.

Abbreviations:
CE Common Era (the equivalent of AD)
BCE Before the Common Era (the equivalent of BC)

This book is dedicated to Yogi Bhajan, whose tireless commitment to sharing the teachings of Kundalini yoga has inspired so many people around the world.

Contents

INTRODUCTION 8

Introduction to Kundalini 8

Yogi Bhajan – A Visionary 11

The Power of Meditation 12

Meditation and Your Well-being 14

Kundalini – A Unique Approach 16

How to Use this Book 18

CHAPTER 1 Awakening Kundalini 20

What is Kundalini? 22

The Origins of Kundalini 24

The Goddess 26

Shiva and Shakti 28

Kundalini in Other Traditions 30

Primal Sound 32

The Subtle Energy System 34

Understanding the Chakras 36

The Chakras and the Endocrine
  System 40

A Gradual Awakening 42

Expanding Awareness 44

CHAPTER 2 Preparing Your Body, Preparing Your Space 46

Getting Started 48

Creating a Meditation Space 50

Purifying the Body 54

Preparing and Eating Food to Aid
  Meditation 56

Tuning in 58

The Art of Listening 60

Overcoming Negative Patterns 62

CHAPTER 3 Prana, Nadis and the Chakras 64

Energy for Life – the Prana Vayus 66

The Flow of Kundalini 68

Body Locks 70

Exercises to Awaken Energy to Prepare
  for Meditation 73

Poses for Meditation and Relaxation 84

CHAPTER 4 The Power of Breath 90

Kundalini and the Breath **92**

The Importance of Pranayama **94**

Developing Breath Awareness **98**

The Navel Centre **102**

Exercises to Master Breath **106**

Circular Breathing **112**

CHAPTER 5 Mantras, Mudras and Yantras 114

Mantras **116**

Seed Syllables **118**

Mudras **120**

Yantras **124**

CHAPTER 6 Meditations for Body, Mind and Spirit 128

Meditation for Emotional Balance
and Intuition **130**

Meditation to Break Habits and Heal
Addictions **132**

Meditation to Release Anger **134**

Meditation for Healing **136**

Meditation to Boost the Immune
System **138**

Meditation for Welcoming Love **140**

Meditation to Lift Depression **142**

Meditation to Awaken Kundalini
and Creativity **144**

Meditation to Create Abundance **146**

Meditation for a Fresh Start **148**

Meditation for Couples **150**

Meditation for Motherhood **152**

Glossary **154**

Further Reading **156**

Index **157**

Acknowledgments **160**

Introduction to Kundalini

Kundalini. This ancient Sanskrit term may conjure up for you all kinds of images and ideas. Mysticism, secrecy, ritual, perhaps even the attainment of bliss or enlightenment. But what exactly is Kundalini? Kundalini practices have been misunderstood for decades in the West, but recently increasing numbers of people have been discovering the benefits of the tradition. Kundalini yoga emerged from the meditative practices of ancient Hindu India, possibly as long as 4,000 years ago, and incorporates a focus on the chakras (the energy centres of the subtle body, see pages 36–9), movement, breathing exercises and chanting. Today, ordinary people are rediscovering Kundalini as a tool to relieve stress, to promote both physical and emotional healing, and ultimately to connect with a profound and transforming spirituality. Kundalini truly has become accessible to everyone.

My own path to Kundalini has been a little unusual. For most of my career I have performed around the world as a professional opera singer. Early on I discovered yoga as a tool to help calm and centre me in the midst of the demands of my singing career. But my first experience of Kundalini took me way beyond the benefits of the type of yoga I had been practising up to that point. I was on a yoga retreat in Chichén Itzà, Mexico, burnt out after a hectic schedule of singing and touring. Intrigued by a form of yoga I knew nothing about, I signed up for a Kundalini class. Deep down I was searching for some inner peace, balance and a greater sense of connectedness through both mind and body. This initial encounter with Kundalini was a very powerful one and I realized during that first class that I had found what I was looking for.

Of course, I didn't immediately surrender my feelings of fear, resistance and doubt about this very different form of practice. However, once I tuned in to the techniques of Kundalini I found a new way of being. The beauty of Kundalini is that it takes you beyond the confusion and clutter of daily life to a

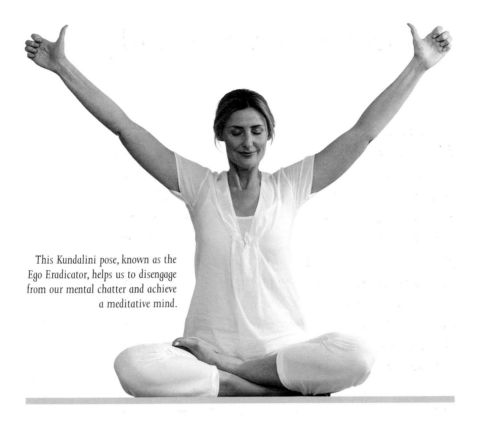

This Kundalini pose, known as the Ego Eradicator, helps us to disengage from our mental chatter and achieve a meditative mind.

place where you experience a sense of real freedom and stillness. At this point the neutral, meditative mind can allow access to inspiration, excitement and new possibilities. Your mind frees itself of the repetitive dialogue of negative voices and confused thoughts – the ancient echoes of the past. The new, raised energetic frequency at which your mind is operating allows you to listen to your mind's authentic voice, the voice of your dreams, passions and purpose. In this neutral space we can accept who we are and embrace all that we are – the light and the shadows, the good and the bad in us.

Today, most people avoid being with their minds in silence. It can seem at the same time both terrifying and lonely. We avoid this experience by distracting ourselves with external stimuli and "busy-ness", to prevent ourselves from going within and developing a conscious relationship with our mind. This helps to create an illusion of feeling safe and in control. But it is in the quiet, still moments that we have the potential to off-load the constant "chatter" and come to a point of peace.

The word "Kundalini" literally means "the coil in the hair of the beloved", and symbolizes the uncoiling of the creative energy that lies dormant at the base of the spine. The image that is often used to describe this energy is of a coiled serpent sleeping. Once we awaken Kundalini energy, we raise our energetic vibration to release stress and allow our mind to come back to peace and balance.

Kundalini meditation combines powerful and effective techniques such as breathing, mudras (hand gestures) and mantras (sacred sounds) to accelerate this process toward a neutral, meditative mind. It is an extraordinarily powerful practice that we can all integrate into our everyday lives. Even if you have only a short amount of time to practise in your day, one Kundalini meditation can bring about real transformation.

In Chapter 6 I have provided a series of Kundalini meditations to address specific issues, such as releasing anger and welcoming love. If you want to commit to a specific meditation for longer than a few days, I would suggest meditating for the same length of time on 40 consecutive days. The number 40 is symbolic – it is often given in ancient scriptures as the length of time needed for enacting change. And your practice will be deepened if you can find a few minutes every day to prepare yourself for meditation with a selection of yoga exercises combined with relaxation poses (see pages 73–83 and 84–89). Start with a minimum of three minutes of meditation if you are a complete beginner, building to 31 minutes if you have the time. For more on how to use this book, see page 18.

Be patient with yourself, as sometimes the benefits of Kundalini meditation aren't obvious straightaway. Keep going and you will eventually notice the changes in ways both subtle and profound. If you are consistent with your practice, you will clear away negative subconscious patterns, replace them with new positive patterns, and transform your life!

Yogi Bhajan – A Visionary

There are different paths to Kundalini. My path was through the teachings of Yogi Bhajan, who brought Kundalini yoga and meditation to the West in 1969. Before that, the techniques of Kundalini as practised in India and Tibet were closely guarded, passed down from master to student.

Yogi Bhajan was born a prince in 1929 in the province of Punjab, in what is now Pakistan. A devout Sikh, it was clear from a young age that he was destined for a spiritual life. He had mastered Kundalini yoga and meditation by the time he was 16 and at the age of 18, when British India was being partitioned into India and Pakistan, he led the inhabitants of his village into India. He completed a master's degree in economics and had a successful career in the Indian civil service. In 1968 he was invited to teach yoga at the University of Toronto, Canada, and in 1969 he moved from there to California. Yogi Bhajan recognized that Kundalini could help the West cope with the increasing pressures of modern life. He offered an alternative to people experimenting with mind-altering drugs, as the sense of connectedness and heightened experience that many were searching for could be accessed through Kundalini.

During his time in the West, Yogi Bhajan built up a legacy of teachings about Kundalini, including over 100 books applying yogic techniques to meditation, drug rehabilitation, healing, rebirthing, business, relationships, psychology and other fields. Yogi Bhajan's intention was "to create teachers not to gather disciples", and he trained thousands of teachers, encouraging them to share his tradition worldwide.

Yogi Bhajan died in 2004 and will be remembered as an inspiring and uplifting teacher with a tireless global vision to help humanity, in his words, "keep up" with the ever-growing demands of the 21st century. This book has been inspired by him, by my teacher Karta Singh and by my deep love of the teachings and my desire to share them with as many people as possible.

The Power of Meditation

I came to Kundalini meditation through my own issues with stress – something that I'm not alone in experiencing. Today, we all face enormous pressures in every aspect of our lives – work, home and relationships. Huge economic, environmental and technological changes are taking place on our planet, and the pace of life is accelerating. We have an overwhelming amount of choice available to us and while this is exciting, it can also feel like information overload. Computers, mobile phones and televisions constantly feed us with information and messages. We are bombarded by radioactive waves emanating from household appliances. All these stimuli affect our minds and our capacity to function at our best. More and more people are suffering from burnout, depression and other psychological problems. But there is one technique that is both accessible to all and effective in counteracting these negative effects – and that is meditation.

Kundalini meditation is a powerful science that can help us to put aside the thoughts that burden the mind, create stress and cause illness in the body. In Western society we have been conditioned to think that the best way to treat depression is with anti-depressant medication, but by being open to healthy, natural alternatives such as meditation, we can come to realize that we no longer have to be slaves to our minds.

Kundalini meditation will help you develop a conscious relationship with your mind, so that instead of being

The Half Lotus pose facilitates the flow of Kundalini energy during meditation.

controlled by your thoughts, you become their master and can eventually remain in a state of elevated consciousness as you go about your everyday life.

The exercises and meditations set out in this book are an opportunity for you to accelerate change. Instead of allowing stress to harm your well-being, you will experience renewed energy levels, giving you the strength, stamina and clarity that are necessary for modern living. You don't need to understand the Kundalini techniques fully to realize their benefits; neither do you need to live a monastic life to experience their power. It is perfectly possible to work them effectively into your ordinary daily life.

As you grow in your Kundalini practice, your mind will become clearer, calmer and less reactive and you will develop a more peaceful relationship with yourself and those around you. Some of these transformations can occur in as short a space of time as 40 seconds, which makes Kundalini practice a highly effective tool for coping with the intensifying energy that we are all experiencing on the planet today. Bringing your thoughts under control may seem like an overwhelming task, but you will discover how to do it. One of the first steps to a meditative mind is bringing the body into stillness. Within that stillness the mind can begin to find its neutral space. When you start to practise Kundalini meditation, you will encounter lots of different and colourful "personas" – facets of your own self, both positive and negative, each with its own agenda. It is your choice to engage or not with them.

Be patient and give yourself time to explore the techniques suggested in this book. Gradually, as you begin to make peace with all the hidden voices that can be buried deep in the subconscious mind – expressing judgment, doubt, fear, confusion, envy and competitiveness – you will shift to a new perspective in which those voices dissipate and you feel more enthusiastic, creative and willing to embrace change and enjoy each moment in your life's journey.

Kundalini meditations can seem strange at first – and there have certainly been times when I myself have been surprised by the instructions – but if you let go of your fears and inhibitions and trust in the process, you will discover how the practice can work for you.

Meditation and Your Well-being

While Kundalini is usually recognized as a largely spiritual practice, there is now medical proof for the many health benefits of meditation for people suffering from chronic pain, anxiety, post-traumatic stress, substance abuse, eating disorders, insomnia, psychosis and many other psychological disorders, as well as for those with terminal illnesses such as cancer.

Scientific studies involving magnetic resonance imaging (MRI) and electroencephalograph (EEG) scans, which allow researchers to observe parts of the brain that are more active than others, have measured the effects of meditation. Neuroscientists observing the brain activity of Tibetan monks with many years of practice in loving-kindness meditation found evidence of significant activity in the insula. Located in the cerebral cortex, the insula helps to monitor emotions and physiological responses such as blood pressure and heart rate, as well as the part of the right side of the brain that is responsible for empathy. This research concluded that we all have the potential to train our minds to become more empathetic and compassionate.

Having visited Tibet and been in the presence of monks and lamas during meditation, I can confirm that the serene calmness and happiness radiating from their minds are reflected in their faces. Just sitting with them and feeling their energetic vibration was a profound and moving experience.

Recent work by the American neuroscientist Professor Richard Davidson, looking specifically at the effect of meditation on the brain, involved the analysis of hundreds of brain scans, as well as asking his subjects to report on their mood. Those scans of people who described themselves as anxious or depressed showed increased activity in the right prefrontal cortex and the area around the amygdalae (the two groups of nuclei involved in emotion-processing). However, in people who were happy and calm, the left prefrontal

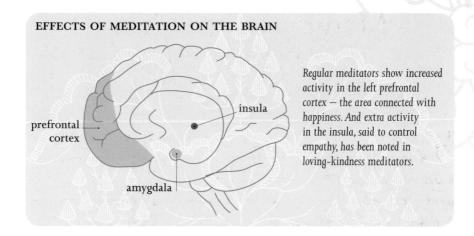

EFFECTS OF MEDITATION ON THE BRAIN

prefrontal cortex

insula

amygdala

Regular meditators show increased activity in the left prefrontal cortex – the area connected with happiness. And extra activity in the insula, said to control empathy, has been noted in loving-kindness meditators.

cortex was the more active area. Davidson concluded from his research that regular meditators were happier than average non-meditators.

Dr Barbara Fredrickson has studied the effect of "loving-kindness" meditation, which requires a focus on feelings of compassion and kindness. Her research found increased positive feelings, improved relationships and reduced depression in meditators, as well as better physical health. Another form of meditation, "mindfulness", which was first developed by Jon Kabat-Zinn in the late 1970s as a stress-reduction programme, has been proven in studies to be effective in helping people with anxiety, chronic pain and fibromyalgia.

In recent studies at the University of California (UCLA), those practising only 11 minutes of Kirtan Kriya meditation (see pages 130–31) every day showed improved short-term memory and cognitive function, and reduced stress levels. This meditation, which uses a Kundalini mantra and mudra (hand gesture), was found to alleviate stress, fatigue and anxiety in adults with memory impairment and in those suffering from Alzheimer's disease.

In my own experience as a professional singer, meditation has helped me enormously in overcoming my pre-performance nerves as well as improving my concentration in preparing for and performing roles. Meditation will help you to strengthen your mind, so that you can guide your body into achieving your dreams, instead of being held back by negative thoughts.

Kundalini – A Unique Approach

Every form of meditation is powerful, but the unique approach of Kundalini makes it especially transformative. It is the combination of five specific elements in Kundalini that is so important. These are: asanas (yoga positions), mudras (hand gestures), bandhas (body locks), breathing and mantras.

Asanas, mudras and bandhas

Many people meditate effectively and powerfully without practising yoga postures, and it is possible to take this approach with Kundalini meditation, too. However, simple body postures known as asanas can allow you to become more tuned in to your body and sensitive to the changes that take place. As Kundalini rises and balances the energy of your body's chakras (see pages 36–9), asanas relating to the major chakras (see pages 73–83) will significantly increase your awareness of your energy levels. For example, Frog Pose (see page 79) is excellent for channelling creative sexual energy in the sacral chakra, while Neck Rolls (see pages 82–3) help you to tune in to the throat chakra, which is associated with our capacity for clear and truthful communication. Any sitting pose where the base of the spine is in contact with the ground is good for creating awareness of the base chakra, such as Half Lotus or Easy Pose (see page 86) or the more demanding Full Lotus.

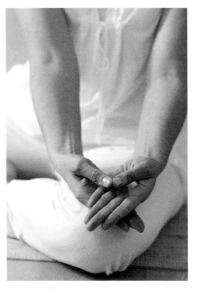

Buddha Mudra helps the meditator to access the neutral, meditative mind.

Mudras are hand gestures that create subtle energetic connections through the nadis (energetic channels, see pages 34–5) to the brain. They can powerfully evoke a spiritual idea or symbol and connect your mind in a very direct way to different parts of your body. The ancient yogis believed the five fingers each symbolized a different human quality, element and planetary influence: for example, the thumb symbolized happiness; the index finger, knowledge; the middle finger, patience; the fourth finger, energy; and the little finger, intuition. Certain mudras, such as Venus Lock and Yoni Mudra (see pages 122 and 123), are very Tantric, balancing male and female energy. The mudras shown in this book (see pages 121–3) can be used in isolation, but will be more powerful when integrated into a specific Kundalini meditation (see Chapter 6).

Bandhas or body locks (see pages 70–72) are used to direct the flow of energy in your body and are key in raising Kundalini.

Breathing

Breathing techniques are another key aspect of Kundalini (see Chapter 4). Yogis traditionally believed that our normal breathing pattern is too rapid and shallow to raise Kundalini energy effectively. Exercises focusing on the regulation of breath play a large part in Kundalini practice, and principally involve slowing down inhalation, holding the breath and then gradually exhaling. In the process we absorb more prana (life-force) and enjoy the physiological and psychological effects of a meditative state.

Mantras

This is the aspect of Kundalini that in many ways interests me the most. As a singer, I find that the chanting of mantras reveals different and fascinating aspects of my voice and mind. The sounds contained in mantras have positive meanings that stimulate energy to clear negativity from the mind (see page 116). In my experience, the sound vibration can be so powerful that the mind is instantly calmed and a feeling of euphoria created. The effect is profound.

When asanas, bandhas, mudras, breathing and mantras are brought together, Kundalini meditation takes you to a new level of awareness and peace.

How to Use This Book

At the beginning of this book I give some background on what we know about the origins of Kundalini and its link to ancient Tantric approaches to spirituality, developed in India many centuries ago. The basic idea of the Tantric approach is that we can all reach a new level of spiritual connectedness through our practices, and through seeing ourselves as microcosms of the energy of the universe. So in Chapter 1 you will learn about some gods and goddesses used as metaphors in Kundalini, as well as the body's subtle energy system (including the chakras) and the sacred power of sound.

Chapter 2 then gets you ready for your Kundalini practice by offering advice on preparing your meditation space, on food and exercises to cleanse your body, and on how to overcome the negative thinking that can block effective meditation practice. Chapter 3 explores the subtle energy system of the body in more detail and explains the energy channels used in Kundalini. In this chapter you will find yoga positions (asanas) and relaxation poses to develop your awareness of Kundalini energy. Chapter 4 focuses on the power of your breath and gives some breathing exercises to help develop control. Chapter 5 looks in depth at some of the key components of Kundalini: mantras, mudras and yantras (sacred diagrams). You will discover how to work with these to enhance your regular Kundalini practice. Finally, Chapter 6 concludes with 12 specific meditations and postures to help heal both body and mind. My hope is that by this stage you will have experienced many of the benefits that come from practising this ancient science.

Some of the meditations include chanting a mantra, and you can download these from my website at www.kathrynmccuskerkundalini.com. Choose a mantra that resonates with you. As you practise the meditations, commit to being with yourself for that time, without distractions. Let your daily practice be your sacred moment, a gift to your body, mind and spirit.

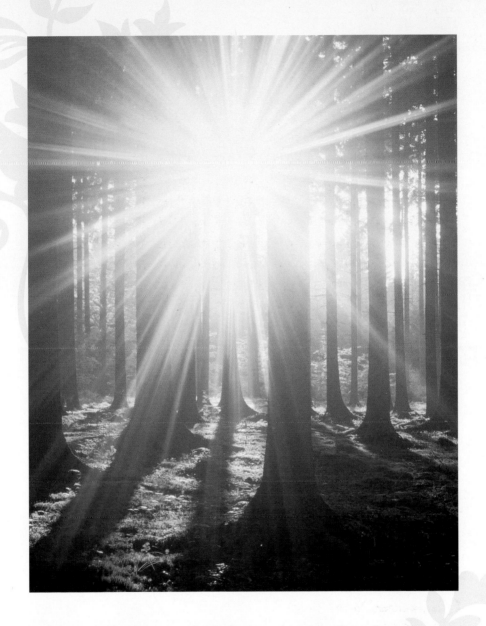

"We can all reach a new level of spiritual connectedness through our practices, and through seeing ourselves as microcosms of the energy of the universe."

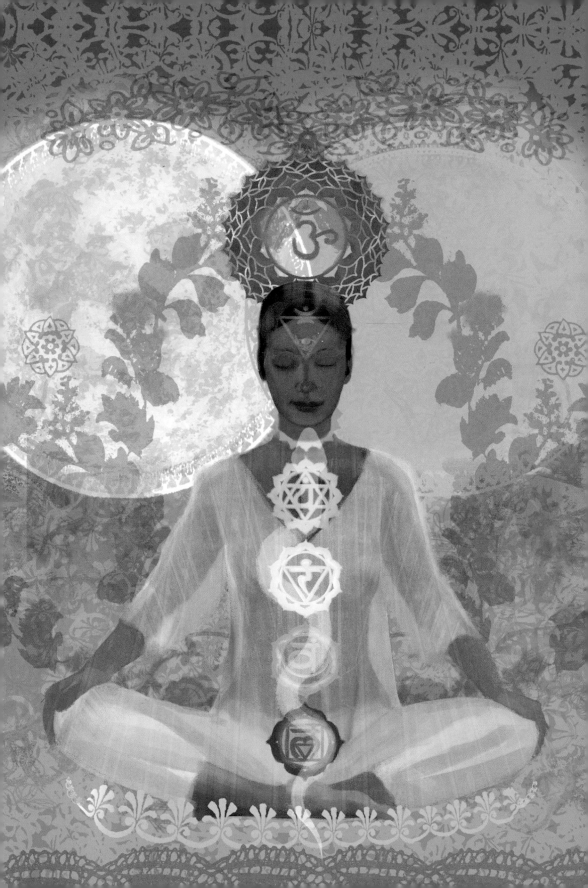

CHAPTER 1

Awakening Kundalini

In this chapter you will discover the ancient origins of this practice and learn about Kundalini in terms of the body's subtle energy system, the primal power of sound and the union of Shiva (male energy) with Shakti (female energy).

"You must be the change you wish to see in the world."

Mahatma Gandhi (1869–1948)

What is Kundalini?

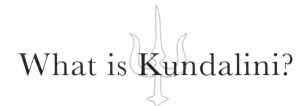

K undalini refers to a special life-force that we are all born with. The term partly derives from the Sanskrit word for "coiled up" or "circular", and Kundalini energy is often described as a coiled serpent that lies dormant at the base of the spine. We can all learn how to activate it.

The experience of Kundalini can expand your awareness, leading to full consciousness. By awakening the energy within us, we can realize our true nature and embrace our full human potential. The purpose of this book is to show you how to do this gradually, safely and naturally (see page 42). You will begin to feel the benefits of your practice and notice real changes in a very short period of time.

Ancient texts describe Kundalini as a female energy, called Shakti, and explain how this energy or power consciousness can rise through the body to unite with pure consciousness in the form of the male Hindu supreme deity, Shiva. In many ways Kundalini yoga can be seen as the uniting of the dualities present in all of us – positive and negative, active and passive, male and female.

Through the practice of Kundalini techniques, this dormant energy is ignited, to rise up through the chakras. In physiological terms (see pages 40–41), this can be explained as the rise of energy up the central column of the spine to the top of the skull where it activates the pineal gland, which sends messages to every cell in the body to relax. When the pineal gland secretes chemicals into the brain we experience a major shift in consciousness. We feel that our body is properly in balance and that we are fully integrated with our reality. We experience a profound peace.

It is not uncommon for people to go through their entire lives without awakening Kundalini; in fact, most people are unaware of the existence of this energy. But anyone who practises some form of yogic discipline, or who has had a genuine spiritual experience, may already have experienced this enormous potential of psychic energy – the body's most powerful thermal current. Why do we want to awaken Kundalini energy? We do so in order to integrate more fully with reality and to realize our full potential. By activating and channelling this energy we raise our consciousness through the chakras, and transform our spiritual awareness into productive action. The gift of Kundalini meditation is the capacity to confront the ego and clear away its attachments, so that you can then listen to your own truth and fulfil your life's purpose.

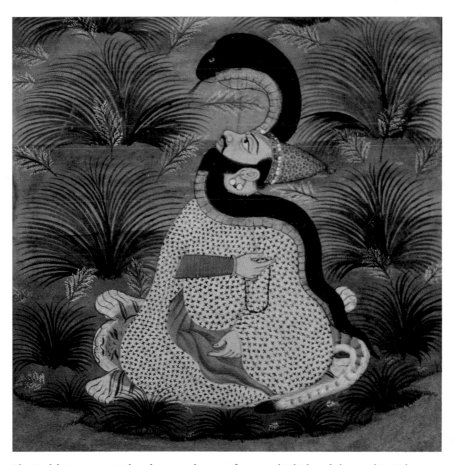

The Kundalini serpent uncoils and rises up the spine of a sage to his highest chakras in this 18th-century Indian miniature.

The Origins of Kundalini

Although it is difficult to be precise about the origins of Kundalini, most of our knowledge comes from the Tantras, a collection of Sanskrit texts probably written down in the 8th century CE, although based on earlier oral traditions dating back to the 5th century. The Tantras were believed to have been revealed by the gods Shiva and Vishnu, and by the Great Goddess, Devi, and transmitted to the world by human sages.

Tantrism seems to have originated in Kashmir and Nepal, but religions throughout India absorbed many of its elements. A key aspect is the belief that the human body is divine and contains within it the hierarchy of the cosmos. This means that through rituals and practice everyone has the potential to achieve spiritual liberation. One Tantric text, the *Ratnasara*, states: "He who realizes the truth of the body can then come to know the truth of the universe."

The Tantric texts all have a common structure of ritual to be observed. This involves purifying the body, creating a divine self through the chanting of sacred sounds or mantras, internal visualization as a type of worship, and external forms of worship such as the use of mudras (hand gestures) and meditating with sacred images such as yantras (visual representations of chakras) and mandalas. The Tantric texts hold that we can all attain bliss through undertaking a spiritual journey, the journey of Kundalini through the body.

It is said that Tantric wisdom can only be passed on by a guru properly initiated into the tradition. The lineage of Kundalini yoga as taught by Yogi Bhajan can be traced back to around 1900 BCE and King Janaka of Mithila, a region now part of Nepal. Originally passed down through the line of kings, this tradition was then passed in the 16th century to Guru Ram Das, the fourth of the 10 Sikh Gurus, who was regarded by Yogi Bhajan as his teacher. When practising the teachings of Yogi Bhajan, we tune in with the Adi Mantra (see pages 58–9) which links us to this Golden Chain of teachers.

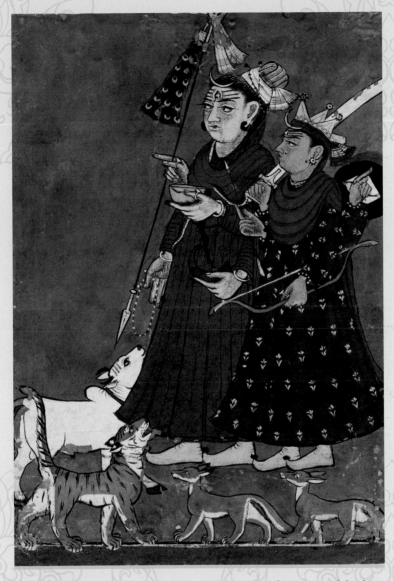

This Indian painting from the mid 18th century shows Shiva discoursing with his divine female counterpart, Devi. The Hindu Tantras usually take the form of a dialogue between Shiva and the Goddess in one of her forms.

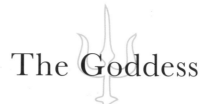

The Goddess

The activation of the feminine principle within us all, the awakening of the Kundalini goddess – Shakti – is a vital part of Kundalini practice. Although the worship of the Great Goddess known as Maha Devi dates back several thousand years or more in India, it was with the rise of Tantrism from the 6th century CE that she was rediscovered and took centre stage.

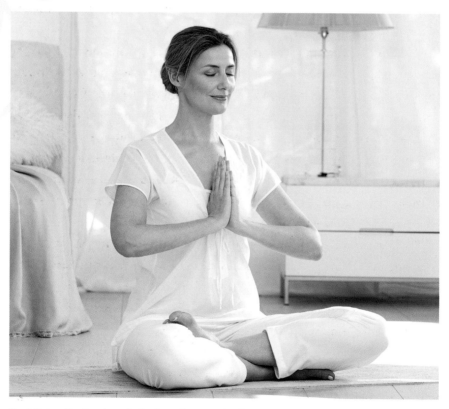

Kundalini meditation channels the divine feminine slumbering within us all – Kundalini Shakti, who lies coiled at the base of the spine.

The different manifestations and roles of Devi in mythology help us to understand the creative power of Kundalini Shakti. Durga represents Devi in her warrior form, the slayer of a great buffalo demon called Mahisa. The god Brahma had granted Mahisa a boon, that he could not be killed by any male, and so the demon thought himself invincible. Yet he is defeated by a female, Durga, who subverts many traditional concepts of the feminine – she is dynamic rather than passive and independent of male authority. Although very beautiful, she is also warlike, heroic and fearless, depicted riding a lion. Ultimately, she pierces Mahisa's chest with a trident and then decapitates him. Durga is praised by the gods for her actions and she promises to help them whenever she is called upon. Her myth is a testament to the female principle as active and powerful.

The Goddess can also adopt the terrifying form of Kali, the Dark One of Hindu mythology, who engages in furious combat on the battlefield or haunts cremation grounds. She is often depicted wearing a necklace of skulls and a girdle of severed arms, symbolizing the karmas (past actions) that she has removed. Kali is important in Tantric traditions as representing everything that normally repels and terrifies us. In Tantrism, resolving dualities is seen as the means of liberation, and hence meditating on Kali allows us to confront the conventional dualities – such as clean and unclean, sacred and profane – that lead to confused perceptions of reality.

The other primary manifestation of the Goddess is as the consorts of the gods, their feminine energies. Sarasvati, the consort of Brahma, Parvati, the consort of Shiva, and Lakshmi, the consort of Vishnu, fall into this category and are models of wifely and maternal devotion. They embody attributes that are more typically "feminine" than those associated with Kali or Durga.

In Tantrism and Kundalini traditions, the Goddess was seen as the ultimate reality – the divine feminine creative power. It is through her that a devotee can be liberated from the cycle of life and death. You may want to focus on a range of manifestations of the Goddess in different traditions during your practice to enhance your awareness of certain chakras (see pages 51–2).

Shiva and Shakti

A nother important concept in Tantrism and Kundalini, related to the theme of the Goddess, is that of integration. In many ancient texts this is seen as an integration of male and female principles, the coming together of the God and the Goddess. In the ancient teachings of the Vedas, the earliest scriptures of Hinduism, the Supreme Being of the universe is pure consciousness, undivided, whole, neither male nor female. However, when pure consciousness manifests itself in the universe it becomes dynamic and forms the world of duality in which we live. The principle of potential action is considered to be the male principle, while action itself and the power and result of that action are considered to be the female principle, known as Shakti. All male deities have a female counterpart, or Shakti, a personification of the energy that takes action in the world.

Throughout India the most important deity is Shiva, the supreme god from whom all life emanates; he is pure consciousness. The ultimate goal of Kundalini practice is to arouse Kundalini Shakti to unite with pure consciousness in the form of Shiva. In this way we can rise above duality and achieve a sense of oneness with the universe. One ancient text, the *Shaiva Purana*, beautifully expresses this unity: "Just as moonbeams cannot be divided from the moon … so Shakti cannot be separated from

Shiva as Ardhanarishvara — half-man, half-woman. This 11th-century statue is from the Chola kingdom of southern India.

Shiva." Each form of energy is vital: Shiva is static energy and Shakti is kinetic energy. Only when the two are combined can creation exist.

One of the most remarkable representations of this idea of male/female unity is the half-male, half-female deity Ardhanarishvara. This deity was actually a manifestation of Shiva as "Lord Who is Half-Woman" and his name literally means "the half of Shiva who is Parvati", Parvati being Shiva's divine consort. Ardhanarishvara was depicted in beautiful sculptures as a half-man, half-woman, one side of the figure featuring the dress and adornment appropriate to Shiva, and the other featuring that of Parvati.

The concepts of male and female union as a means to attaining liberation were also celebrated in sacred poetry. The 12th-century *Gita Govinda*, the "Love Song of the Dark Lord", celebrates the love between Krishna and Radha and is seen as an allegory of the soul's craving to merge with the Divine.

Kundalini and sexual energy

Because Kundalini involves the union of female and male energies, your sexual experiences are likely to be heightened as you work with Kundalini energy. Kundalini is concerned with the development of awareness and understanding in every aspect of life, and sexuality is no exception.

All the exercises and meditations in this book work with the concept of integrating female and male energy. By removing blocks and cleansing the subconscious mind, we can experience the essential nature and qualities of the male and female polarities. And with the integration of the two parts of our being, we begin to see our real self with more clarity. This energetic union, which is a sort of alchemy, can be achieved at the heart chakra (see page 37).

"Coiled like a snake, Kundalini lies in its latent form.
Whoever causes this Shakti to move shall find liberation."

Hatha Yoga Pradipika (3:108)

Kundalini in Other Traditions

Although Kundalini is primarily Hindu in origin, other traditions also believe personal liberation to be possible through accessing the divine within yourself. One key aspect of the Vajrayana or Tantric Buddhism that developed around the 7th century CE was the use of ritual in the enlightenment process. "Vajra" is a Sanksrit term translated as "diamond" or "thunderbolt", but its wider meaning describes everything that is unfaltering, unchangeable and brilliant. The vajra was often depicted in art as a sceptre-like object with a spherical centre representing Buddhist reality or shunyata, the absolute emptiness from which all matter emerges. Its identical ends symbolize the union of such apparently dualistic concepts as male/female, permanence/impermanence. The vajra is often held by a deity as a symbol of wisdom, with another deity holding a bell, symbol of compassion. The combination of these two principles was believed to be the key to awakening.

A key practice in Vajrayana is meditating on one's identity with the divine, on one's own "Buddha nature". As the Dalai Lama said, "The body of a Buddha is attained by meditating on it." This is another aspect of non-dualism, one of the key points of Tantric and Kundalini practice. When we are aware of the divine within ourselves, we see that there are no opposites in life; all is one.

Vajrayana Buddhism embodied this idea in the primordial Adi-Buddha and his consort, who are the union of compassion (selfless action) and wisdom (direct awareness of reality). The female stood for wisdom; the male, for compassion. Many Buddhist artworks depict an Adi-Buddha couple, tenderly embracing, representing the inseparable nature of male and female.

OPPOSITE *This 13th-century thangka (scroll painting) from Tibet depicts the Adi-Buddha Vajrasattva with his consort Sattvavajri, the female wisdom principle.*

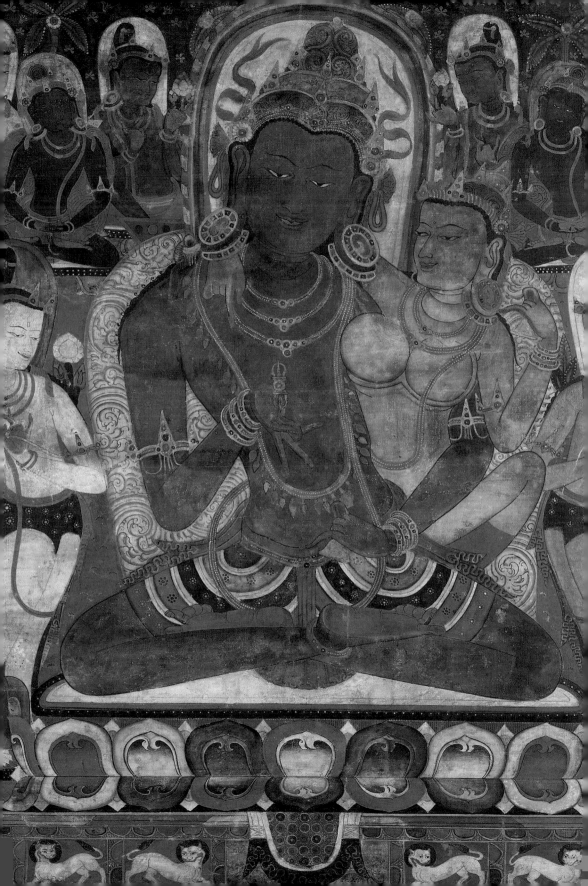

Primal Sound

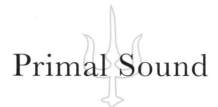

Sound is of particular importance in Kundalini traditions, and the chanting of sacred sounds or mantras is a key element in Kundalini practice. Later in the book (see page 116), I explain in more detail what mantras are and provide some examples that you can practise yourself, but first I want to explain a little more about the transformational aspects of sound.

In Hinduism and Buddhism, the sound AUM or OM is considered to be the start and end point of creation. It is believed that mystics can hear the vibration of the cosmos – a gentle humming of the atoms of the universe. The Sanskrit term for this is anahada nada, which means "sound produced without striking"; this cosmic hum is the pulsating vibration of the universal energy. AUM or OM represents this sound and is highly sacred.

Each part of AUM or OM is rich with meaning. This sound is composed of three parts, "AH", "OH" and "M", and refers, in the Hindu tradition, to the trinity of creation, preservation and destruction (Brahma, Vishnu and Shiva). The sound of AUM instantly produces positive vibrations and takes the listener to a state of mental stillness. Chanting AUM will help you to calm your mind, settle your thought processes and realize your true self.

In Kundalini yoga as taught by Yogi Bhajan, we tune in with a Gurmukhi mantra that begins with the sound ONG. This sound vibration aligns us with our creative path and connects us to the eternal sound of the universe.

Both AUM and ONG have strong vibratory effects. While AUM refers to the force of all creation, ONG refers to the Creator, who is the Doer of all action. ONG makes things happen and generates Shakti, the creative and generative force of life (see pages 28–9).

The sound ONG should be vibrated in the nasal passages and the centre of the head, and its vibration should be felt in the body's lower chakras (subtle energy centres, see pages 36–9), especially the second or sacral chakra. This

OPENING THE CHAKRAS WITH SOUND

You can use a specific mantra and mudra (hand gesture) to open each of the seven major chakras (see pages 36–8) to the flow of energy. As you practise, try sitting in a Half Lotus or Easy Pose (see page 86). When chanting these mantras, note that "A" is pronounced "ah" and "M" as in the "ng" of "king".

TO OPEN THE ROOT CHAKRA Bring your hands into Gyan Mudra (see page 121), on top of your knees. Focus on the root chakra and chant LAM.

TO OPEN THE SACRAL CHAKRA Bring your hands into Venus Lock (see page 122), at the level of your ovaries/testes. Focus on the sacral chakra and chant VAM.

TO OPEN THE SOLAR PLEXUS CHAKRA Bring your hands into Yoni Mudra (see page 123), at your navel. Focus on the solar plexus chakra and chant RAM.

TO OPEN THE HEART CHAKRA Bring your hands into Prayer Mudra (see page 121), at your heart, in the centre of your chest. Focus on the heart chakra and chant YAM.

TO OPEN THE THROAT CHAKRA Bring your hands into Lotus Mudra (see page 123), at your throat. Focus on the throat chakra and chant HAM.

TO OPEN THE THIRD EYE CHAKRA Bring your hands into Buddha Mudra (see page 122), in your lap. Focus on the third eye chakra and chant ONG or AUM.

TO OPEN THE CROWN CHAKRA Bring your hands into Gyan Mudra (see page 121), on top of your knees. Focus on the crown chakra and chant NG or AH.

powerful vibration also activates the pituitary gland, which is connected to the third eye chakra (see page 40). The third eye chakra has a powerful relationship with the sacral chakra. Together, they can give us the power to be creative, manifest our dreams and make an active contribution to the world.

Sound is thus a spiritually charged phenomenon and helps us to approach ultimate reality most closely. That is why mantras underpin so much of our Kundalini practice.

The Subtle Energy System

To understand how Kundalini energy works you also need to understand your subtle energy system. Ancient texts held that, in addition to our physical body, we also have a "subtle" body that is not visible in the ordinary sense, but is nevertheless a powerful energetic system. Some texts stated that as many as five subtle energy sheaths surround the physical body. These sheaths or layers help us to connect with universal energy, as each sheath is linked not only to this infinite energetic flow, but also to the body's chakras. The word "chakra" comes from the Sanskrit for "wheel", conveying the sense of a centre of whirling energy. There are many chakras within the body, but the seven major chakras are the ones used most often in energy healing and can be most easily located as they are positioned roughly along the spine of the physical body. These chakras are particularly important in Kundalini meditation as Kundalini activates each of the seven major chakras in turn as it rises through the body. Chakras are looked at in detail on pages 36–9.

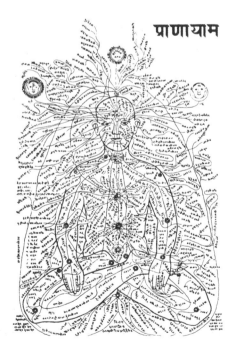

प्राणायाम

The sheaths of the subtle body relate to our physical body via energy channels called nadis. The term "nadi" derives from the Sanskrit for "motion" or "vibration". Although

This is a traditional Indian representation of the body's web of nadis — so complex is this network, it would be impossible to map it accurately.

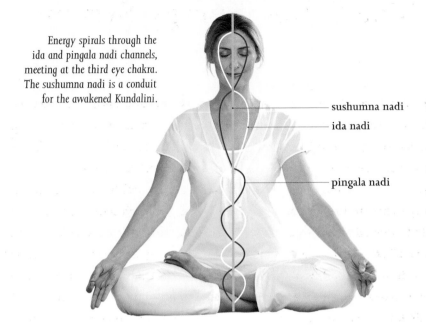

Energy spirals through the ida and pingala nadi channels, meeting at the third eye chakra. The sushumna nadi is a conduit for the awakened Kundalini.

sushumna nadi
ida nadi

pingala nadi

there are thousands of nadis running through the body, Kundalini yoga focuses on three in particular: the sushumna, the ida and the pingala.

The sushumna nadi runs up the centre of the spine, from just below the base chakra to the crown chakra. Within sushumna are three more channels called vajra, chitrini and brahmani. It is through the brahmani nadi that Kundalini energy moves upward when it is finally awakened.

On either side of sushumna flow the two other important nadis. On the left is the white "moon" or female nadi called ida, while on the right is pingala, which is known as the red "sun" or male nadi. Energy flows through these two channels from the base of the spine, spiralling in opposite directions around the central sushumna channel, which finally meets these two nadis at a point between the eyebrows. The sushumna channel remains closed at its base until the moment when Kundalini is awakened and begins to flow upward. When we breathe, chant or meditate, we are not only calming the mind, but also nourishing the nadis and the whole subtle body.

Understanding the Chakras

Developing your awareness of the energetic function of each of the chakras is important in helping to understand how Kundalini energy works as it travels through your body. Each chakra has an important function and is correlated with different aspects of our lives, affecting our perceptions, feelings and choices. The seven major chakras interact with, and influence, our thoughts, moods and health.

Through Kundalini exercises and meditation we can explore the mysteries of the chakras, bringing to light ways in which we are blocked, and learning techniques to release our inner energy and full potential.

All the chakras are interconnected and work in unison. The first three major chakras are sometimes known as the "lower triangle" and are connected to the physical needs of the body and of life. The other four major chakras, or the "upper triangle", work with our spiritual and universal consciousness.

The chakras are usually depicted as lotus flowers. The Kundalini opening or awakening of each chakra can be seen as the awakening of consciousness within ourselves.

Base or muladhara chakra

Also known as the root chakra, the first chakra is located at the base of the spine and is where the Kundalini energy lies dormant. This chakra's element is earth. It connects us to the physical world, and is the foundation of our physicality and bodily well-being. All our fears, habits and addictions can be trapped in the base chakra. When it is unbalanced or blocked, this can manifest in a lack of self-worth, and in distrust and insecurity. When this chakra is balanced and cleared, we feel a renewed sense of self-worth and an acceptance of who we are.

Sacral or svadhisthana chakra

The second chakra is located at the site of the sexual organs and the third and fourth spinal vertebrae. It is associated with change and its element, water, reflects its qualities – flow and flexibility in life. This chakra controls sex, reproduction and mental creativity. People balanced in this chakra are creative and have a passion for life. They usually have a healthy sex life and are aware of their generative power to pass on life. An imbalance of energy in this chakra can create an unhealthy obsession with sex or indulgent fantasies, leaving us feeling empty, shameful and guilty.

Solar plexus or manipura chakra

Also known as the navel chakra, the third chakra is situated in the area of the solar plexus, navel and digestive system. Its element is fire. Here we explore our personal power and how we use our will – to empower ourselves or to control others? When this chakra is balanced, your navel centre is strong and you have good physical health. You take the initiative and have the courage to succeed. Imbalances here manifest as excessive greed, a drive for personal power and an attitude of "What's in it for me?".

Heart or anahata chakra

This chakra is located at the "heart centre" of the body, in the centre of the chest. The heart chakra is the balance point between our physical self and the higher levels of spiritual consciousness. When we open the heart chakra, we can experience true love. It is here that we can reconcile the physical and the emotional with the spiritual. This chakra relates to kindness, compassion and selfless giving. A person balanced here will be in harmony with other people and nature. If the energy here is out of balance and blocked, we act from our emotions and feelings. This can manifest as giving and sharing with those who do not deserve it or want it, leaving us feeling lonely and rejected, and questioning the existence of love.

Throat or vishuddha chakra

Located at the throat, the fifth chakra is associated with sound and communication. Its element is ether, a subtle, heavenly energy. From here we vocalize our truth and monitor our words. When this chakra is open and strong, our words have power and we communicate effectively. This chakra has particular importance for chanting mantras, and by meditating on it we become aware of how sound can heighten our spiritual experience. If there is an imbalance here you may be highly opinionated or too blunt, or you may be unable to express yourself effectively.

Third eye or ajna chakra

Also known as the brow chakra, the sixth chakra is located just above and between the eyebrows. It is the site of our direct connection to the infinite source of wisdom – the place we often focus on in meditation and where intellect meets intuition. Through our third eye we begin to sense a higher consciousness beyond time and duality. This is where ida and pingala unite with sushumna. Regular meditation combining breathing and mantras can activate this chakra, increasing your intuition and focus. When this chakra is blocked you will feel a sense of confusion about what is real and lose faith in your connection to the universe.

Crown or sahasrara chakra

At the top of the skull, the seventh chakra is the "Thousand-Petalled Lotus". Here we realize that we are all One, total awareness is achieved and all polarities are integrated. When Kundalini energy is raised here, we connect to our higher self, to the universe and to the Infinite. A person open in this chakra will know a reality beyond the physical senses. If this chakra is blocked you may doubt spirituality and lose faith in the greater whole.

OPPOSITE *A practitioner of yoga, painted in India in the 18th century. Chakras are represented by lotus emblems and depictions of Hindu divinities.*

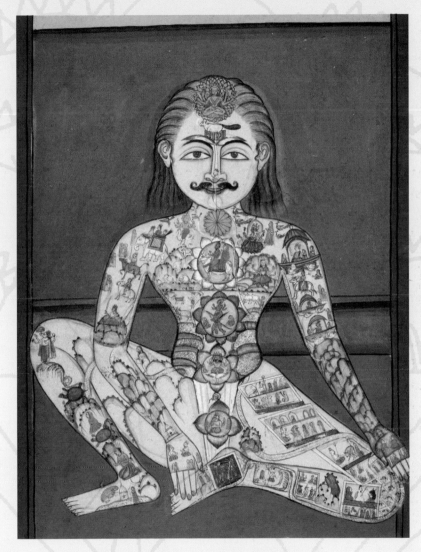

"No man is free who is not master of himself."

Epictetus (55–135 CE)

The Chakras and the Endocrine System

It has often been observed that the positions of the chakras correspond to some of the principal glands in the body's endocrine system. Whether ancient masters intuitively understood this is unknown, but many people today believe that this relationship is significant and that working with your chakras is not just beneficial to your psychological, emotional and spiritual development; it can also help you to achieve optimum physical health.

Each of the subtle body's seven major chakras corresponds to an important site in the endocrine system of the physical body.

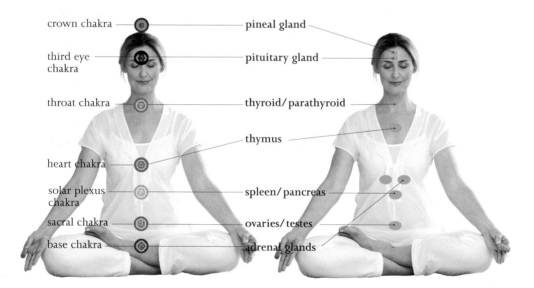

crown chakra — pineal gland

third eye chakra — pituitary gland

throat chakra — thyroid/parathyroid

thymus

heart chakra

solar plexus chakra — spleen/pancreas

sacral chakra — ovaries/testes

base chakra — adrenal glands

The endocrine system

Governing our hormones, our body's endocrine system is vital for healthy functioning. Hormones regulate our metabolism, growth, development and tissue function, and can also have a big influence on our mood.

Linked to the base chakra, the adrenal glands sit near the kidneys and are chiefly responsible for releasing the hormones associated with stress, as well as affecting kidney function.

The reproductive glands control our reproductive function, and are associated with the sacral chakra.

The pancreas, linked to the solar plexus chakra, produces digestive enzymes vital in absorbing food.

The thymus, associated with the heart chakra, plays an important role in the immune system.

The thyroid controls how quickly the body uses energy and makes protein, and affects sensitivity to other hormones. It is linked to the throat chakra.

The pituitary gland, linked to the third eye chakra, is crucial in many functions including growth, blood pressure, aspects of pregnancy and childbirth; it also produces endorphins associated with pain relief and mood.

The pineal is the least understood yet perhaps the most interesting of the glands. It seems to play a role in the production of melatonin (the hormone responsible for regulating our sleeping and waking patterns), and to affect the development of the reproductive glands. Because the pineal is located deep within the brain, many people have speculated that it must be of fundamental importance to humans. It is traditionally linked to the crown chakra.

A Gradual Awakening

A major misconception in the West regarding Kundalini is that it can be a dangerous practice. In 1970 the Indian Kundalini practitioner Gopi Krishna (1903–1984) wrote *Kundalini: The Evolutionary Energy in Man*, in which he described his own sudden awakening. Gopi Krishna undertook arduous daily meditation for many years until, at the age of 34, he had a startling moment of profound awareness, which he described in his autobiography as the effect of Kundalini energy rising through him to transform his consciousness.

Although this book did much to popularize the concept of Kundalini, it also led to concerns that the sudden development of awareness when an individual was insufficiently prepared could be alarming. The key point in all Kundalini practice is to develop awareness of your internal energy in all its aspects. Meditating on the qualities of each chakra in turn is an important way in which the different aspects of your psyche can be integrated. The aim is not to rush headlong to the goal of total awareness and enlightenment, but rather to gain wisdom and understanding from all the energies of your psyche.

The great psychologist Carl Jung studied the passage of Kundalini through the chakras and saw it as a process by which the psyche becomes whole, in which the functions of thinking, feeling, sensing and intuiting are reconciled and balanced. This means that each stage of the journey of Kundalini through the chakras is an important point at which to pause and absorb its meaning. Far from the focus being on the achievement of a great rush of energy up the spine, the process should be about a gradually growing awareness and a resolving of tensions and energetic blocks. As with any discipline, problems arise when we expect instant results without practice and understanding.

OPPOSITE *Work steadily, calmly and patiently with Kundalini and new awareness will come to you naturally and safely.*

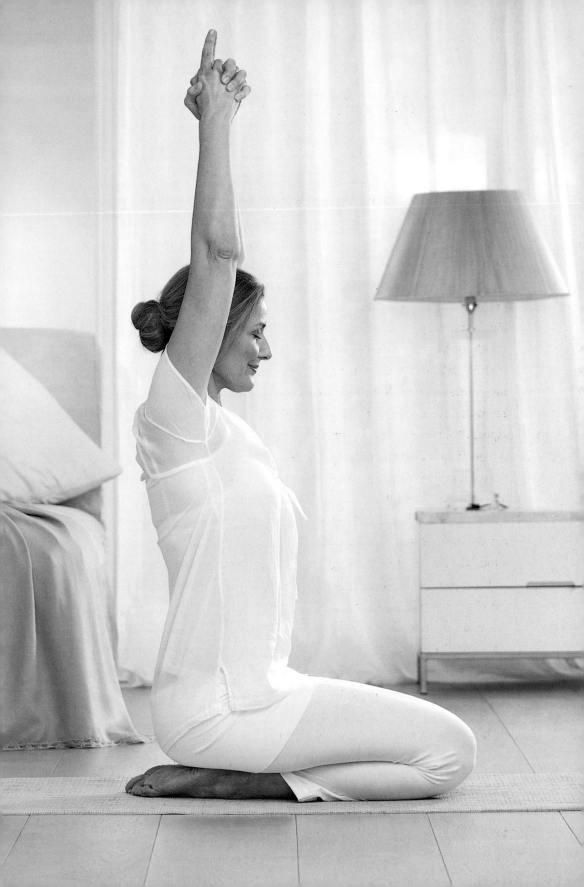

Expanding Awareness

Kundalini energy is the awakened identity of your true self, which can be experienced as a timeless and infinite love of the soul. Kundalini is a complete science that may be divided into different components, yet it is the experience of participating in the totality of that structure that allows you to touch something beyond the physical body and recognize the infinite quality of the soul. In the moment when Kundalini is awakened, the ego has nothing to do. There is only bliss, joy and a huge sense of gratitude for that which has been given as a gift to all of us.

The total experience of a Kundalini awakening can have a profound effect on your awareness of your mind, body and spirit. The transformative power of the awakened Kundalini releases blocks and overcomes difficulties, opening paths to healing and change. Kundalini energy has the capacity to cut rapidly through the limitations of the ego, so that you can tune in to your innate wisdom and true potential. There are no words that can capture the experience.

The human mind has the potential to be creative and expansive, but in practical reality we don't train our minds to take part in this process. Through regular Kundalini meditation you can awaken Kundalini energy and release the mind's control. Training the mind in this way and giving it a regular experience of its infinite potential will free up the creativity of your intellect and the intelligence of your soul.

Once Kundalini energy is raised, it can cleanse the subconscious mind of all the different elements that become trapped there – fears, phobias, unfulfilled desires and dreams. Once released, our thoughts become lighter and clearer and we can then begin to understand how to train our minds to realize peace, prosperity and health at all times.

It takes time, patience and commitment to discipline the mind, but even a few minutes a day can create a good habit and establish a path to expanding

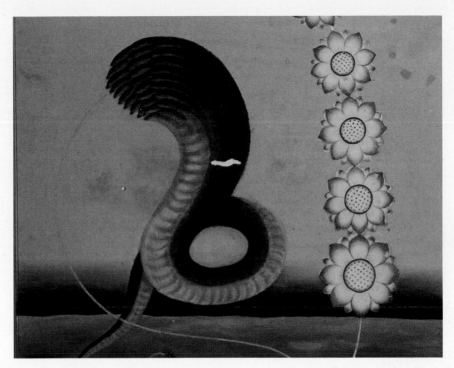

Detail of a 19th-century Rajasthani painting showing the Kundalini serpent rising through the chakras, which are symbolized by lotus flowers.

awareness. This book will give you the techniques to learn how to develop your intuition and work toward a neutral mind, so that you recognize what is real and important to you.

We all experience challenges and stresses in our everyday life, and the key to rising above those pressures is to develop a more meditative mind. If everyone desired a neutral, calm and intuitive mind, imagine how much happier humanity would be!

With a more balanced mind, life's challenges don't seem so overwhelming and one is able to trust that the difficult times will pass. Awareness creates clarity and a knowingness that life is about successes and failures and that it is possible to embrace it all. Kundalini can help you to achieve a clear and intuitive mind to help you to face these challenges.

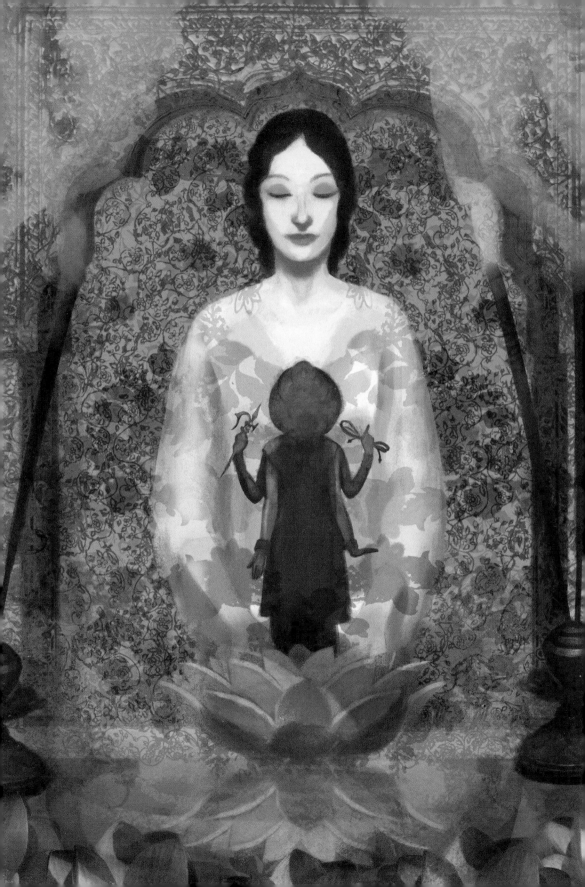

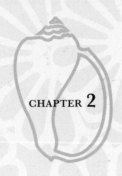

CHAPTER 2

Preparing Your Body, Preparing Your Space

This chapter helps you to prepare for your Kundalini
practice by purifying your body and personal space, and
working on some of the emotional and psychological
barriers that may inhibit your development.

"Meditation is the life of the soul; action, the soul of meditation.
And honour the reward of action."

Francis Quarles (1592–1644)

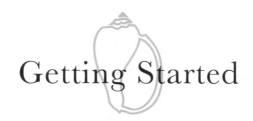

Getting Started

So often our mind creates excuses! Instead of embracing a lifestyle that truly supports and nourishes us, we distract ourselves with a mantra that goes something like: "I know I should have, but ...."

Setting up healthy habits, and having the courage and commitment to keep on with them, requires a feeling of "Yes, I can!" This is usually sensed in the stomach, as a "gut feeling", which inspires you to initiate a course of action and then follow it through.

Students often tell me that they don't have time in their lives for regular meditation practice, but simply by saying "Yes" and starting, you can free yourself from the control of such negative thinking. And with time this initial impetus will be reinforced by your experience of the many emotional, physical and spiritual benefits that come from looking after your mind.

Any of the meditations and exercises suggested in this book can easily be incorporated into your day. If you are a complete beginner with meditation, I would recommend dedicating at least three minutes a day to your practice, working with a specific meditation or exercise for 40 days. For those who are more experienced, I would suggest 20 minutes or more every day for at least 40 days. Having the confidence to begin will fire your enthusiasm and you will notice how changes start to filter through into your everyday life. Your thoughts will become clearer and calmer and you will trust more in life's flow. This new awareness will help you to cope more easily with everyday pressures.

There are a number of things you can do to make the healthy habit of daily Kundalini practice feel more creative and fun, such as setting up your own meditation space (see pages 50–51). Preparing such a space, and purifying your body through cleansing, grooming and diet (see pages 54–7), will not only help to focus your mind, but also give a ritual feel to your practice, deepening your experience.

FINDING INSPIRATION

One of the best ways to encourage your practice is to join a Kundalini class with an experienced teacher who can guide you in your journey. The group consciousness will support and inspire you. To get you thinking, here are just a few inspiring experiences from my own students and colleagues:

- "I had a lot of resistance to the meditations and chanting, but something inside resonated. I started going to classes regularly and my journey led me to the teacher-training in France. I have embraced the meditation, and recently completed a meditation to heal my relationship with my father. I feel I have managed to release a lot of anger and confusion buried deep inside me. I have become more comfortable with who I am and attract more positivity into my life – it's been truly amazing!" (*Martha, artist and art teacher*)

- "Kundalini was integral to my healing after my life crumbled when I discovered my partner was having an affair. I was given a meditation to practise daily and, as I continued, I found my depression lifting and my emotional state balancing." (*Hannah, psychology MA and photographer*)

- "Kundalini played a key part in my recovery from the repetitive strain injury that threatened to end my musical career. Through intensive study of Kundalini yoga and other techniques, such as the Alexander Technique, I succeeded in getting rid of the original injury and overcame many other problems in the process, such as deep insecurities and creative blocks." (*Matt, violist, violinist and composer*)

- "I have worked in financial markets since the 80s and experienced all the associated extremes in personal behaviour. Finding Kundalini yoga was a turning point in my life. I attended many Kundalini classes and amazing things started to happen. My energy levels and stamina increased, and I also tuned into self-awareness and intuition. I am now able to approach life in a more calm, pro-active manner. The beauty of Kundalini is that it takes you back to the real you, free of preconditioned patterns of behaviour, and gives you a deeper sense of purpose and connection." (*Simon, financial broker, Kundalini teacher and co-founder at Alchemy Centre, London*)

Creating a Meditation Space

In many parts of the world, a shrine or sacred space is a vital part of the family home. For example, in most homes in India a small shrine, separate from the rest of the house, is maintained as a focus for meditation and worship. The shrine, which may be kept on a shelf or in a cupboard, often contains an icon or statue of a particular deity to whom offerings of food, flowers and incense are made. The offering of light (aarti) is often also important in these domestic ceremonies. It is believed that by bringing a camphor lamp toward the icon or statue, and then moving the light back toward the devotee, the warmth and light of the deity are transported to the individual.

Decorations such as flowers and candles will give your meditation space a special atmosphere. In time, your space will come to feel a part of you and be a constant reminder of your commitment to yourself.

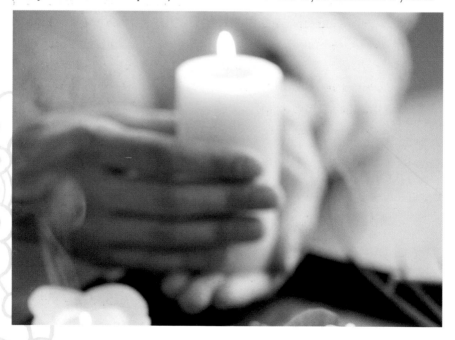

CREATING YOUR OWN MEDITATION SPACE

Even if you don't have much room, try to set aside a small, quiet corner for meditation. Having such a dedicated space will encourage you in your practice.

- On a small altar, arrange a candle and some decorations that are meaningful to you, such as photos or flowers – anything that uplifts and inspires you.

- If you feel it's appropriate, you could include a small statue or an image to represent the Goddess in one of her manifestations.

- Place a yoga mat or a cushion on the floor, so that you can sit comfortably.

- Include a shawl or a blanket to keep you warm.

- If possible, ask the people who share your home to reserve this small space for you alone.

Using goddesses

As we saw earlier (see pages 26–7), the Goddess can take many forms. Each of the following different incarnations of the Goddess is believed by some yogis to have a special connection with one of the seven major chakras. As an alternative approach to the use of primal sound in opening chakras (explained on page 33), you might like to consider these goddesses when targeting a specific chakra in your Kundalini practice, and perhaps choose one of them to use as a focal statue or icon in your sacred space.

Devi The Great Goddess, the ultimate source of all things and the feminine principle. As Kundalini is a female energy and located at the base of your spine, focus on Devi when you are meditating on your base chakra.

Radha The beautiful consort of Krishna, who falls passionately in love with him and he with her. Their sensuous love story is told in the famous poem *Gita Govinda*. You may like to meditate on Radha as you focus on your second chakra, the sacral chakra, which is linked with your sexuality.

Durga A great warrior goddess – beautiful, powerful and famous for slaying the buffalo demon, Mahisa. Durga is often shown seated on or attended by a lion or a tiger. You may wish to focus on her as you search for inner strength and courage during meditation on your third chakra, the solar plexus chakra, your place of will-power.

Parvati The name of this manifestation of the Goddess means "Daughter of the Mountain". Considered to be the most beautiful woman on earth, Parvati fell madly in love with Shiva. She won him as a husband because of her ascetic discipline, and their marriage became a model of happy conjugal love. You might like to focus on Parvati when you are meditating on your fourth chakra, the heart chakra.

Sarasvati The goddess of speech, learning, the arts, science and music. She is often shown seated on a lotus playing a string instrument called a vina. As you meditate on your fifth chakra, the throat chakra, which is associated with communication, you may like to visualize Sarasvati.

Tara This goddess is beloved throughout the Indo-Himalayan Buddhist world. The name "Tara" means both "Star Lady" and "She Who Carries Across" or "Saviouress". This popular deity guides people who are struggling on their spiritual path and offers compassion and liberation to them. She is a wonderful goddess to focus on whenever you are meditating on your sixth chakra, the third eye or brow chakra, connected to your intuition.

Prajnaparamita This is the Buddhist goddess of supreme, transcendental wisdom. Prajnaparamita, whose name means "Perfection of Wisdom", is the ultimate teacher and the eternal mother. She is most appropriate for work on the highest of the seven chakras, the crown chakra.

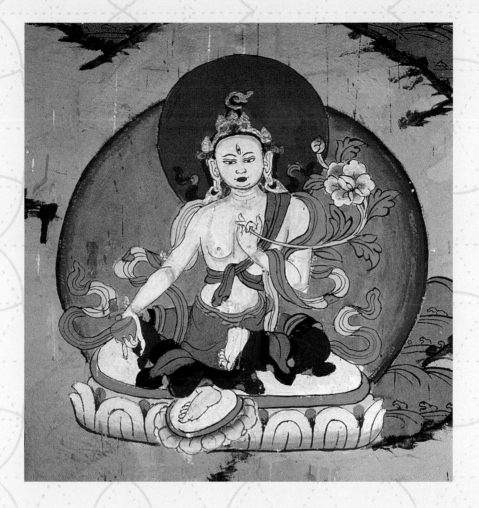

"O universal mother, with perfect understanding, full of compassion,
You came into being for the liberation of the world
O Tara, you are luminous, with beautiful eyes, joy of starlight,
Brimming with pity for all beings, saviour of us all;
Blessed lady, see me and all living things as your children ...
O mother, saviour, guardian, remover of all obstacles, homage to you!"

The Hundred and Eight Praises of Tara

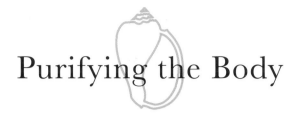

Purifying the Body

A central aspect of ritual in many traditions is the importance of purity, and ideally all forms of worship and meditation should be practised when the individual is as free from pollution as possible. This means cleansing and grooming the body so that you are ready to begin your practice fresh and untainted by the material world. In Kundalini we normally try to do our sadhana (daily spiritual practice) in the early hours, sometimes before the sun rises. This quiet time is good for meditating and cleansing the mind. I definitely notice a difference in the quality of my day when I meditate before dawn. If you have never experienced getting up at this time, try it at least once!

Traditionally, Tantric practitioners (called tantrikas) would practise nyasa and mudras before beginning their Kundalini yoga practice. Nyasa, or the sensitizing of the body by the gentle touch of the fingertips, is believed to awaken the body and make it ready for meditation practice. Mudras, or hand gestures (see pages 120–23), signify a person' readiness for the divine to enter sacred space.

Cleansing ritual is important in many cultures. Native American traditions, for example, featured the sweat lodge, a kind of sauna that cleanses toxins from the body. Smudge sticks and herbs were also lit to cleanse space, and some tribes practised "going to water", bathing in the moving water of rivers.

Before your Kundalini practice in the morning, I recommend taking a cold shower for 1–3 minutes, as this hydrotherapy opens the capillaries and cleanses the body's toxins. If you find this challenging, try massaging your body with pure oil first, to give your skin a protective coating. If you allow yourself time to adjust to the cold water, your body temperature will regulate and you will feel awakened and invigorated, ready to embrace the day. You may also like to burn some incense or sage to cleanse your meditation space, or chant a mantra to set your mind in motion and free it from everyday thoughts.

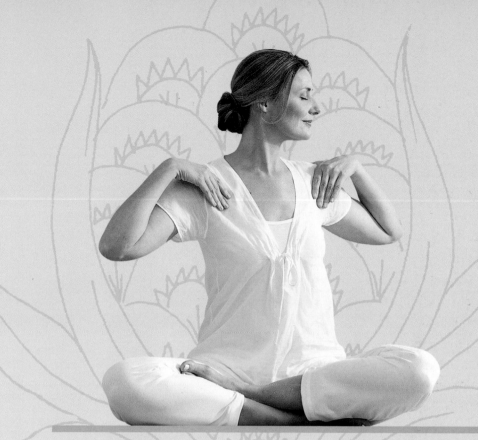

When meditating, I prefer to wear white – the colour of purity.

CLOTHING

Whether you prefer to meditate in the morning or in the evening, it is good to change your clothing so that you prepare yourself physically and mentally for your sacred time. Getting dressed focuses the mind and reminds you that you are about to do something special. It is a different feeling jumping out of bed and meditating in your pyjamas than it is meditating in clothing that uplifts and inspires you.

I prefer to wear white, natural, organic cotton when I practise yoga and meditate. It is believed that lighter colours have a positive effect on your aura, and white in essence symbolizes purity. I definitely feel lighter and calmer when I wear white – but the choice is yours.

Preparing and Eating Food to Aid Meditation

Being mindful of what you eat and how you eat is a meditation in itself. Combining meditation with food and exercise gives you three ways in which you can take responsibility for your health.

Eating consciously requires self-discipline, patience and commitment, but when you begin to experience the benefits for your mind and body, you will start to eat more intuitively, paying attention to what supports you physically, mentally and spiritually. Over the years, my diet has become more finely tuned through trial and error. I now know my body and mind prefer simple, light and nourishing vegetarian foods, especially when I am regularly meditating and practising yoga. As you go deeper into your meditation practice, you too will find yourself drawn to foods that enhance your clarity of consciousness, such as meals made with fresh vegetables and fruit.

It is important to discover for yourself which foods support your health. Food should never be an obsessive, self-destructive pleasure. If you remember that food contributes to your prana (life-force), which fuels body and mind, you will be encouraged to explore foods that are fresh, energy-giving and preferably organic. Try to source foods that are locally produced as they are fresher than food flown in from thousands of miles away. You will really be able to taste the difference!

According to the traditional Indian health system, Ayurveda, certain foods are especially good for the body, and also lead to greater clarity, harmony and balance of mind. These are the sattvic or pure foods, and from time to time you might want to consider following a diet based purely on these, say for a week while you take your Kundalini practice deeper. Sattvic foods include fresh fruit and vegetables, salads, fruit juices and nuts, such as almonds, pine nuts and walnuts, as well as seeds such as sesame, pumpkin and flax. Most

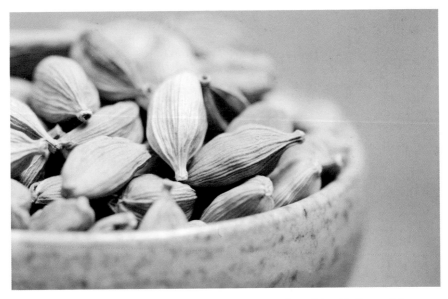

Cardamom is one of the spices considered sattvic or pure in Ayurveda, traditional Indian medicine.

mild vegetables are considered sattvic, however pungent vegetables such as chilli, garlic and onion are categorized as more rajasic, referring to a quality of mind that induces energy and action. Wholegrains such as rice, whole wheat, spelt, oatmeal and barley are all recommended, as well as legumes including mung beans, lentils, split peas, chickpeas (garbanzos), tofu (beancurd) and bean sprouts. Sattvic spices are mild, and include basil, cardamom, cinnamon, coriander (cilantro), cumin, fennel, fenugreek, fresh ginger and turmeric.

Not only are the ingredients important to your health, so too are the ways in which they are prepared and served. Try to prepare food with mindful awareness and gratitude. I often enjoy singing a mantra when I prepare a meal, as I find this relaxes me and creates a positive vibration to support the digestive process. Before eating, take a few moments to meditate on and appreciate your food. Savour each mouthful so that it produces maximum nourishment.

Try to eat three light meals a day, and avoid eating late at night as it takes at least three hours to digest your food. Your sleep will improve and you will feel clearer and calmer when you rise to begin your meditation practice.

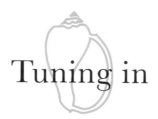

Tuning in

Whenever you feel that you need to centre yourself, or before you begin a Kundalini exercise or meditation, it is helpful to "tune in" with a Kundalini mantra. The sound vibration prepares and focuses the mind and body and calms the parasympathetic (unconscious) nervous system. Immediately, you will feel a deeper sense of connectedness and peace.

ONG NAMO GURU DEV NAMO

In Kundalini we tune in with a specific mantra made up of ancient sounds – ONG NAMO GURU DEV NAMO. This mantra is known as the Adi (primal) Mantra and creates a link to the spiritual masters of Kundalini. These sounds come from the Gurmukhi language, and by vibrating them we are calling for guidance, creating a union between ourselves and our higher self.

ONG is a variation on the cosmic syllable AUM or OM and invokes the infinite creative energy. NAMO (pronounced "nah moh") has a similar meaning to the word namaste, "I bow to you". When we chant them together, they mean "I bow to the infinite creative energy." GURU is the inner teacher who helps us make the transformation from darkness to light. DEV (pronounced like "Dave") means "transparent", and GURU DEV NAMO chanted together is a call to the divine teacher within and to universal wisdom.

1 To begin chanting, sit in Half Lotus or Easy Pose (see page 86), with your eyes closed. Press your palms together in Prayer Mudra (see page 121), creating a pressure with your thumb joints at your sternum.

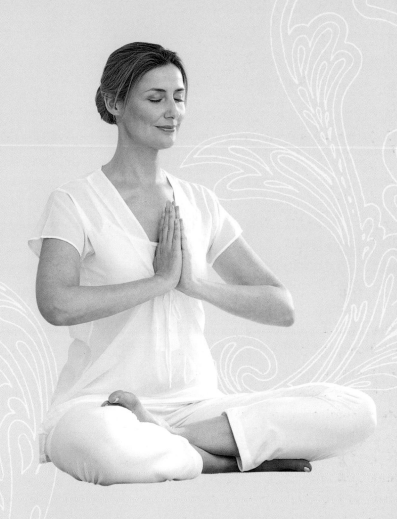

2 Take a deep breath and chant the whole mantra in one breath, or chant ONG
   NAMO, then take a half-breath and chant GURU DEV NAMO. Slightly pull
   the navel in as you chant ONG and feel the vibration behind the nose. The
   first syllable of GURU is short and the second is long. The "R" is rolled at the
   roof of the mouth to activate reflex points that connect to the hypothalamus,
   pineal and pituitary glands, to neutralize your mind.

3 Chant the mantra three times or continue to repeat it for as long as you feel
   you would like to.

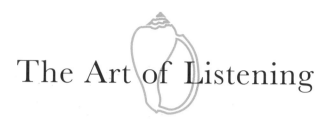

The Art of Listening

It is no wonder that we find it a challenge to really listen when our daily life is consumed by changing focus. Whether it's our mobile phone, email, radio or TV, the constant demands on us to read, speak, write or listen are distractions that prevent us from deep listening. Yet deep listening is vital for inner peace. We are all searching for inner stillness and calm, but until we begin to slow down, reflect, become present and cultivate silence, we will struggle to realize the art of listening. One of the keys to listening more deeply is a daily practice of meditation. When we are still and quiet, we create space to listen to that all-knowing intuitive voice within us that has all the answers.

We choose whether we wish to listen, but most of the time we are unaware that we are making that choice. When we discover that we have consciously chosen to listen, fear and doubt drop away and we begin to trust the guidance of our soul.

Being comfortable with silence will help to transform your capacity to listen, so take the time to be quiet and simply be. Meditations that integrate breath and mantras will help you to manage different energy states (both physical and emotional) and they will support you in cultivating silence.

Deep listening occurs at the heart level, which requires a trust within you. When you open up to love, you will begin to feel more expansive and more connected.

The following are some simple practices you can do each day to help you to slow down, reflect, become present and listen deeply:

- Spend at least a minute in silence every day.
- Take a deep cleansing breath before you respond to anyone, including yourself. Get to know yourself so you can listen to your soul.
- Be mindful of each moment, becoming more aware of your relationship with yourself and with those around you.

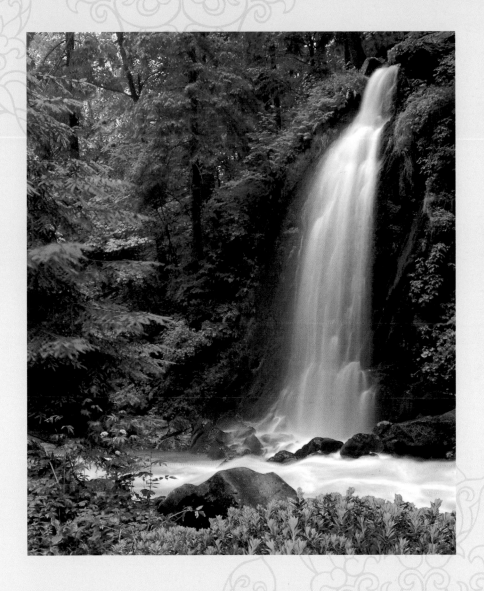

"When we are still and quiet, we create space to listen to that all-knowing intuitive voice within us that has all the answers."

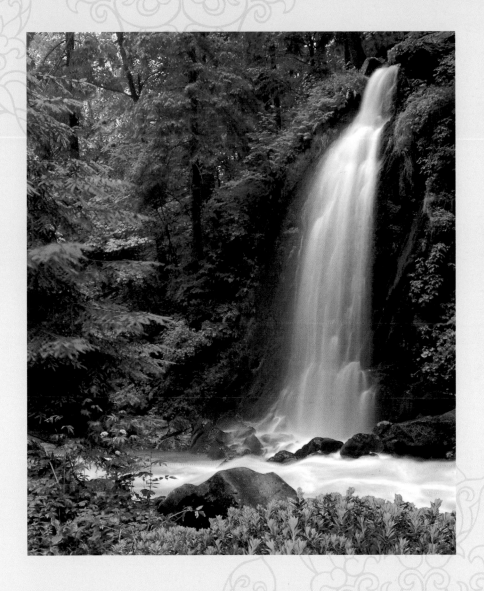

Overcoming Negative Patterns

The intellect is continually releasing thousands of thoughts, but only some of these thoughts become emotions. Everybody has emotions; they are essential for us to live as social animals. Our emotions can enter the subconscious in a confused and turbulent way or they can be transformed in a pure and loving way.

When emotions are all-consuming, they become dangerous. I have witnessed so many students stuck in self-destructive patterns of behaviour as a result of their emotions holding them back. Chaotic, disturbing emotions can create patterns that start to dictate our lives and become habits that are difficult to break. When confused emotions become habitual, we are unhappy and life seems painful. If we meditate, we can break those negative patterns, purify the mind and live more in the moment.

Trust in the process

It is hard to learn anything when the ego controls us. How many of us have created chaos and drama in our lives, reacting without really knowing why? There are very few people who don't have a habit of one kind or another. Some habits make us happy and joyful while others make us unhappy and sabotage our life. Many habits are formed in childhood and we can then spend a lot of our adult life playing out our neuroses. A bad habit can be difficult to break – the ego justifies it and we then feel a false sense of empowerment in having it. But over time the habit becomes exhausting and debilitating and eventually we start to see that it isn't really creating joy or helping us to realize our true potential in life.

The learning comes when we cleanse the subconscious enough to receive wisdom, knowledge and inspiration. Through a daily practice of meditation, a new, good habit is created. Destructive emotions embedded in our subconscious dissolve and the ego melts away. We then trust more in our intuition and less in the chaotic emotions that have fuelled our ego. All those emotions that once seemed important and meaningful are released, and slowly we begin to see the freedom, beauty and joy in life again.

Experience the joy of letting go

Allowing time for silence, emptiness and quietness gives us a new perspective on life, but this is not usually the attitude of people in the Western world. I find myself consciously having to create time to be in silence as there are so many distractions. Many people feel selfish, guilty or lazy about taking time out from their busy day, but if you allow yourself a few minutes off from the "daily grind", you will begin to see the stresses and strains of life disappearing and experience gratitude unfolding.

It is challenging sometimes to find the work and rest balance. Kundalini can remind you of that balance as the meditations and exercises in this book work directly with the yin (female, receiving) and yang (masculine, action) energy in the body and mind.

One of my most powerful meditation experiences was the first meditation given to me by my first Kundalini teacher – the meditation was called Sodarshan Chakra Kriya (see Meditation for a Fresh Start, pages 148–9). I and 35 other students were told to practise this extremely powerful meditation for 31 minutes on 40 consecutive days. Most of us had never done a Kundalini meditation for that length of time, so you can imagine our reaction! It was a huge learning experience for us all and each and every one of us went through a life transformation. The meditation confronted us with our ego and all our human emotions. After two weeks of battling with the meditation, I let go and trusted in the process. I then noticed a profound shift. The negative thoughts and destructive emotions began to disappear and by the end of the 40 days I experienced an overwhelming sense of calm, peace and gratitude. It was at this moment that I realized how powerful and transformative meditation can be!

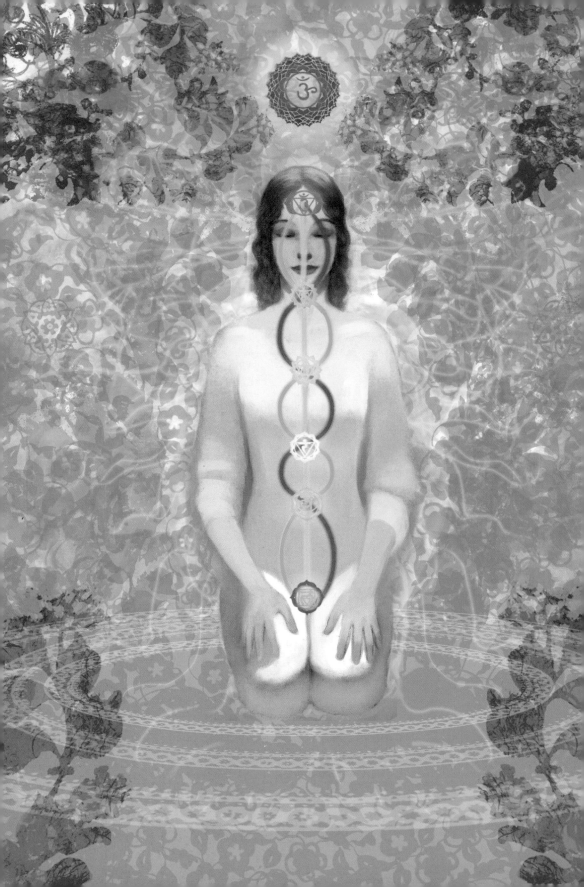

CHAPTER 3

Prana, Nadis and the Chakras

Prana is the life-force, the energy of the universe. When
prana flows properly through the nadis, we have the
capacity to awaken Kundalini, balance the chakras and
bring the mind and body back into a state of true
joy and real peace.

"In this cage [body] there are 72,000 nadis. Of these, the
sushumna nadi gives rise to great delight in yogis."

Hatha Yoga Pradipika (4:18)

Energy for Life –
the Prana Vayus

Kundalini helps us to gain awareness of prana, the subtle life-force, the energy we breathe through the mind and the body. Prana travels through the body, dividing itself into five different rhythms and frequencies called prana vayus. The five main prana vayus are: apana, samana, udana, vyana and one also called, a little confusingly, prana. If there is too much or too little of a particular prana vayu, then physical, mental or emotional imbalances can occur.

Techniques combining movement, breathing and mantras, as well as the way we eat and act, help to bring the prana vayus back into their natural rhythm and flow. When they are in balance we have a sense of stillness, flexibility and intuitive awareness. In this state we sense not only the rhythm of our soul, but also that of the entire universe. By using Kundalini techniques appropriately, you will find that you become more sensitive to the flow of prana, so that you can balance your emotions and increase your mental capacity.

Each of the prana vayus has a different location and function in the body.

Apana vayu

Apana has its home below the navel and is connected to all the functions relating to elimination through the rectum, bladder, colon and genitals. These days we need powerful apana to eliminate the increasing amount of toxins we receive from our environment. Apana will also assist you in knowing what you need to retain and what you need to release. When your apana is strong, you will have a sense of security and the capacity to move forward.

Samana vayu

Samana moves between the chest region and the navel and controls much of the body's metabolism. Strong samana gives emotional clarity and discernment.

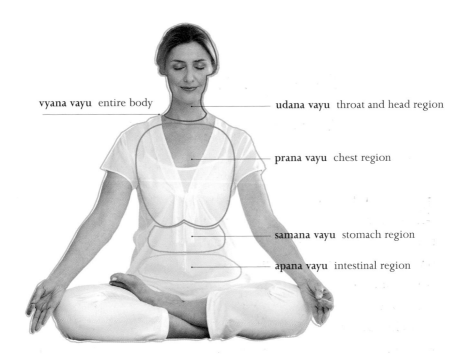

vyana vayu entire body

udana vayu throat and head region

prana vayu chest region

samana vayu stomach region

apana vayu intestinal region

Prana vayu

Prana gathers between the neck and the base of the chest. This energy is linked to inspiration and the healthy functioning of the lungs. When the rhythm of prana is strong, the lungs will feel expanded and you will be charged with energy and ready for life. You will breathe with openness and your mind will be positive.

Udana vayu

Udana lies in the larynx and the head. It is opposite to prana in that it projects air upward and outward. It is actively involved in all forms of speech. With strong udana you will have powerful projection and communication skills.

Vyana vayu

Vyana moves through the entire body and is subtle in its rhythm. It controls the body's coordination of muscles and joints, and helps integration and connection. If vyana is strong, you experience a sense of inter-connectedness and flow.

The Flow of Kundalini

One of the key processes in opening your body up to the flow of Kundalini is to strengthen prana and apana. If these two energies are balanced, the other prana vayus should adjust in turn.

Balancing energy flow

The channels through which prana flows around the body are called nadis, and they are similar in some ways to the meridians of acupuncture. They are connected to one another via the chakras. As we saw in Chapter 1, three nadis are particularly important to understanding the flow of Kundalini:

- Ida nadi is on the left of the spinal column. The ida represents the negatively charged energy (apana) or lunar energy, which eliminates body wastes and has a calming, cooling and restorative effect upon the body and mind.
- Pingala nadi is on the right of the spinal column. It carries positively charged energy (prana), which has an energizing and heat-producing effect.
- Sushumna nadi is in the centre of the spinal column. This is the primary channel in Kundalini and is also known as the "Silver Cord".

Once you have activated the sushumna nadi and opened it to Kundalini, you have the potential to activate all 72,000 nadis. There are several techniques that will help you do this, one of the most powerful being mantras (sound vibrations). Choose a meditation that includes a mantra from Chapter 6 and feel the sound vibrating through your spine as you chant.

Kundalini energy lies dormant at the centre of the base of the spine, where the sushumna originates. Kundalini will not awaken and rise until the two energies – prana (positive) and apana (negative) – are integrated and balanced in the base chakra.

Raising Kundalini

Pressure is required to raise Kundalini up the sushumna. Through a combination of the Root Lock (see page 70) and inhalation, prana is directed down to the solar plexus chakra, while apana, through the Root Lock and exhalation, is drawn upward to the solar plexus chakra. The meeting and uniting of the two forces create a powerful heat in the solar plexus chakra, which lights up the sushumna. With breath control, mental focus and the Root Lock, the integrated energies leave the solar plexus chakra and descend to the base chakra, where they stimulate Kundalini. Breath control and the Diaphragm and Neck Locks (see pages 71–72) cause Kundalini energy to spiral up the sushumna to the third eye and crown chakras, making a double loop at the throat chakra, then flowing back down through the chakras to its starting point. To effectively raise Kundalini, certain blocks and toxins must first be cleared from the nerves, energy channels and chakras. Breathing techniques and mantras, combined with certain postures (see pages 73–83), will help with the cleansing process.

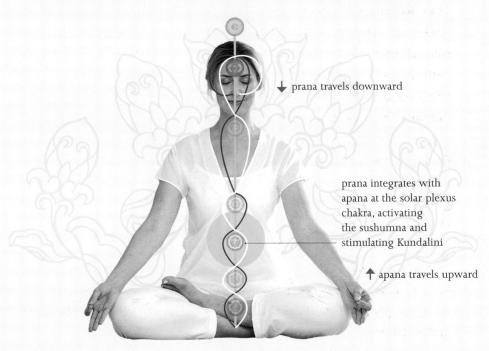

↓ prana travels downward

prana integrates with apana at the solar plexus chakra, activating the sushumna and stimulating Kundalini

↑ apana travels upward

Body Locks

Body locks, known as bandhas, are specific combinations of contracted muscles within the body. By using these locks effectively, you can direct the flow of prana and apana into the main energy channels involved in the awakening of Kundalini energy. Applying locks will help you to maximize the effects of your pranic life-force, enabling changes in nerve pressure, blood circulation and the flow of cerebrospinal fluid. All the locks help to consolidate the body's energy to increase awareness and self-healing.

The three most important locks are Root Lock (Mul Bandha), Diaphragm Lock (Uddiyana Bandha) and Neck Lock (Jalandhara Bandha). When applied together these three locks are called the Great Lock (Maha Bandha).

ROOT LOCK

The Root Lock or Mul Bandha is frequently used when raising Kundalini energy at the base of the spine. Mul means "root" or "source" and this lock's function is to unite the two main energy flows – prana and apana – at the navel so that Kundalini energy can awaken. The Root Lock becomes stronger with practice and may be applied at the end of the energizing exercises (see pages 73–83) and the meditations in Chapter 6.

1 Sit in Rock Pose (see page 87) with a straight spine and exhale completely. (This lock can also be applied after inhaling fully.)

2 Activate the lock by contracting the anal muscles and sexual organs inward and upward toward the navel point. At the same time, pull your navel in toward the spine.

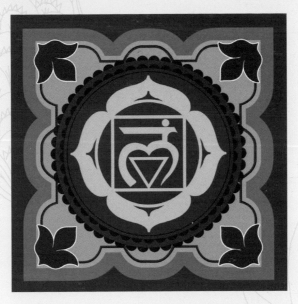

Representation of the base or muladhara chakra, also known as the root chakra, which is activated by the root lock.

DIAPHRAGM LOCK

The Diaphragm Lock or Uddiyana Bandha gently massages the heart muscles and intestines. It supports the flow of prana through the central nerve channel of the spine and up into the neck area. It also helps to support the functioning of the hypothalamus, pituitary and adrenal glands. If you regularly practise the Diaphragm Lock, you will feel more joy, vitality and compassion. From my own experience as a singer, I know that it has increased my breathing capacity and created a more open and free vocal expression.

1 Sit in Rock Pose (see page 87) with a straight spine and exhale completely.

2 Lift the diaphragm up and back as far into the chest cavity as possible. At the same time contract the abdominal muscles toward the spine.

CAUTION: If applied forcefully on the inhalation, the lock may increase pressure in the heart, blood and eyes.

Neck Lock

The Neck Lock or Jalandhara Bandha is generally applied in all chanting meditations and breathing exercises. It helps to balance and stimulate the thyroid and parathyroid glands, activating the higher functions of the pituitary gland and potentially the pineal gland. This lock helps to direct the flow of pranic energy into the upper areas of the brain stem and also regulates the pressure created through some powerful Kundalini meditations.

1 Sit in Rock Pose (see page 87) with a straight spine and exhale completely.

2 Lift your chest and sternum up and at the same time gently stretch the back of your neck by pulling your chin toward the back of your neck. Keep your head level and centred without tilting it forward. Your neck and throat muscles remain loose and you should feel your chin relax between the two collar bones.

Great Lock

The Great Lock or Maha Bandha is the name given to all three locks when applied at once. When this happens the nerves and glands are rejuvenated, creating a feeling of harmony. The blood can then circulate into the reproductive glands, nourishing the male and female sexual organs.

1 Sit in Rock Pose (see page 87) with a straight spine and exhale completely.

2 Apply all three locks: start with the Root Lock, then add the Diaphragm Lock, followed by the Neck Lock.

PRANA, NADIS AND THE CHAKRAS

Exercises to Awaken Energy to Prepare for Meditation

The following postures, also known as asanas, prepare the body for meditation and assist with cleansing blocks and toxins within the body. They can easily be slotted into your daily life, are suitable for all levels of experience and can be practised at any time of the day. You may want to do them separately or in sequence for one or two minutes each. As you practise, spinal fluid will gradually begin to circulate and you will feel more flexible, balanced and energized. Each movement combined with pranayama (breathing, see Chapter 4) will distribute prana throughout the body and you will feel the beneficial effects immediately. Practise each exercise with your mouth and eyes closed, and inhale and exhale through your nostrils. Roll your eyes gently upward and inward toward your third eye – midway between your eyebrows – as this helps to develop a meditative mind and allows you to go deeper into the experience.

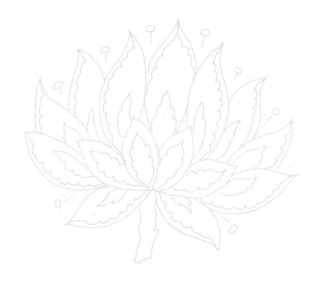

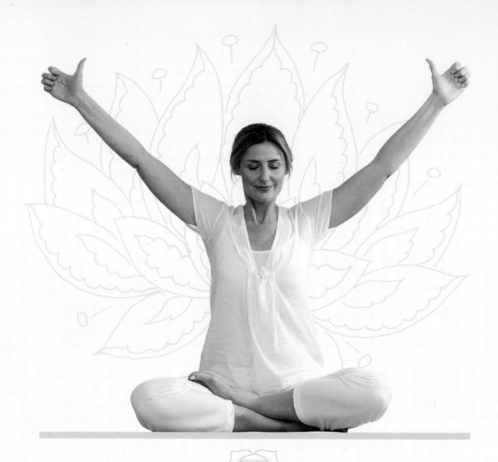

EGO ERADICATOR

In this exercise your thumb represents your ego or personal psyche, which is transformed and balanced, helping you to achieve a neutral mind. This exercise stimulates the solar plexus, heart, third eye and crown chakras.

1 Sit in Half Lotus or Easy Pose (see page 86) and curl your fingertips onto the pads of the palms, keeping your thumbs at right-angles to your palms.

2 Raise your arms at 60° to the sides of your body and do Breath of Fire (see page 107) for 1–3 minutes.

3 To finish, inhale and touch your thumbs above your head. Breathe out and stretch your arms down on both sides of your body. Relax and feel energized, alert and centred.

SPINAL FLEXES

This exercise works on the lower part of the spine where Kundalini energy is stored, stimulating the base chakra.

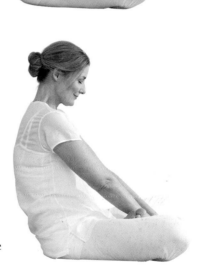

1   Sit in Half Lotus or Easy Pose (see page 86).

2   Take hold of your ankles with both hands and inhale deeply as you flex your spine forward.

3   Open your chest and lift your ribcage, keeping your shoulders relaxed and open.

4   Exhale and focus on slowly rounding your spine, bringing your shoulders forward. Keep your head parallel to the ground. Start slowly and gradually increase the pace as you flex your spine back and forward, synchronizing movement and breath. Repeat for 1–3 minutes.

5   Come back to the centre and inhale deeply. Hold your breath and apply Root Lock (see page 70).

6   Keep squeezing your muscles as you bring your chin slightly inward and imagine drawing energy up your spine.

7   Hold for about 30 seconds and then exhale and relax your breath and the pose.

SUFI GRINDS

Sufi Grinds help to clear blocks and bring your body and mind back into balance, stimulating the base, sacral and solar plexus chakras. They encourage the channelling of Kundalini energy from the lower spine upward, and help to strengthen the digestive system and the muscles in the back and waist.

1 Sitting in Half Lotus or Easy Pose (see page 86), place your hands firmly on your knees.

2 As you inhale begin to rotate your spine forward in a clockwise direction, rolling through your hips and waist, creating a circle. Feel yourself "grinding" from the base of your spine, as you keep your head relatively still and your heart centre open. Do not drop your head down.

3 As you rotate your body back and around to the left and front, begin to exhale. Continue for 1–2 minutes.

4 Now reverse the direction, so you are inhaling in an anti-clockwise, circular movement. Exhale as you come around to the right and back to the front. Allow yourself to go deeper into the circular movement as though you were dancing your spine. Feel yourself becoming one with the breath and the movement. Continue for 1–2 minutes.

5 Come back to the centre and inhale deeply, applying Root Lock (see page 70). Visualize energy rising through the chakras.

6 After about 30 seconds, relax and release the pose.

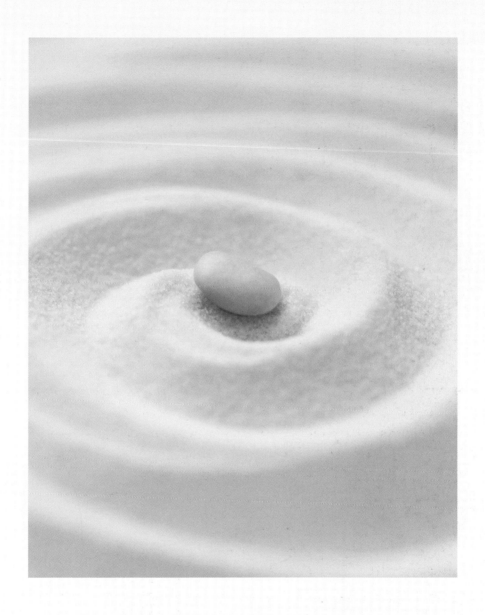

"Allow yourself to go deeper into the circular movement as though you were dancing your spine. Feel yourself becoming one with the breath and the movement."

LIVE NERVE STRETCH

This exercise stimulates the base chakra. It loosens the lower spine, hips and thigh muscles, stretches the sciatic nerve and increases flexibility.

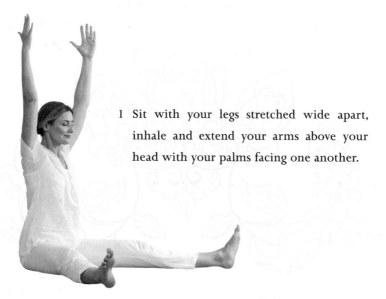

1 Sit with your legs stretched wide apart, inhale and extend your arms above your head with your palms facing one another.

2 Exhale, reach your arms down your left leg and, if you can, grasp the toes of your left foot. If you can't, stretch down as far as you can.

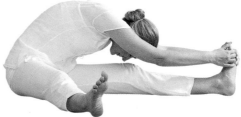

3 Inhale straight up to the starting position and exhale, reaching down your right leg. If you can, grasp the toes of your right foot.

4 Repeat for 1–3 minutes.

FROG POSE

This position is excellent for activating apana in the first three chakras: the base, sacral and solar plexus chakras. It will increase your sexual and creative energy, and build inner strength and stamina. Practising Frog Pose will also circulate energy to the heart and the higher chakras. If you are lacking inspiration and motivation, and need the courage to let go and trust, then practise this pose regularly.

1 Squat on your toes and bring your heels together. Spread out the soles of your feet, just like a frog.

2 With your hands on the floor and your arms between the knees, try to keep your upper body as straight as possible.

3 Close your eyes and focus them at the third eye, between your eyebrows.

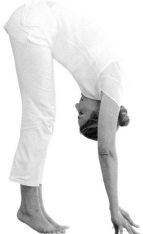

4 Inhale as you straighten your legs, raising your hips while trying to keep your heels off the ground and your hands on the ground.

5 Exhale as you bend your knees and return to the squat position.

6 Continue for up to 26 repetitions, building up momentum as you go and releasing any fears or frustrations.

7 Relax for 2–5 minutes in Baby Pose (see page 87).

Cow and Cat

These two poses are great for increasing flexibility in your spine as well as stimulating the main nerves in the cervical vertebrae. This exercise will circulate spinal fluid and integrate energy throughout the spine. If practised after Frog Pose, it will increase the transformation of sexual and digestive energy from the sacral and solar plexus chakras into the higher centres of the spine. With regular practice, you will notice how flexible your spine becomes; this will not only help you physically, but also allow you to take a more flexible approach in general to your life.

1 Kneel, with your hands on the ground shoulder-width apart and your knees below your hips.

2 Keeping your elbows straight, inhale through your nose, bringing your head up and bending your spine toward the ground (Cow).

3 Close your eyes, rolling them up toward your third eye.

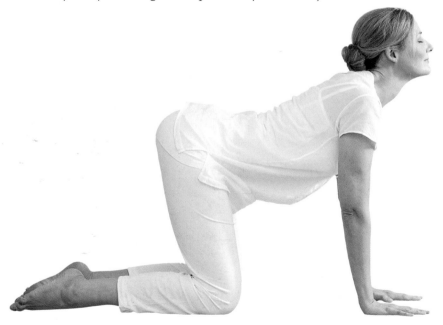

4 Exhale through your nose, flexing your spine in the opposite direction so that your back is arched upward, bringing your head down and tucking your chin in toward your chest (Cat).

5 Continue, alternating between Cow and Cat for 1–3 minutes with a rhythmic and powerful breath through the nose. As you feel your spine becoming more flexible, gradually increase your speed. Imagine you are dancing and breathing through your spine.

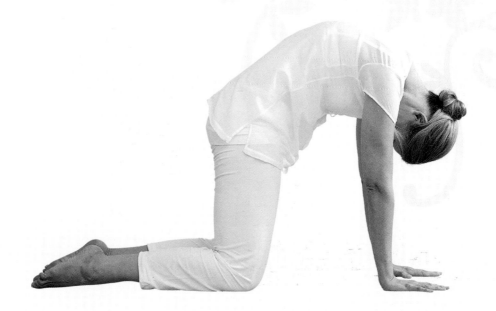

NECK ROLLS

Neck Rolls are a simple and effective way to release tension in the neck muscles and increase blood flow to the brain. This exercise stimulates the thyroid, parathyroid, pituitary and pineal glands, which are responsible for releasing hormones and creating health and harmony in the entire body. Neck Rolls are good for completing the energy-awakening sequence.

1 Sitting in Half Lotus or Easy Pose (see page 86), begin rolling your head in a clockwise circular motion, bringing your right ear toward your right shoulder.

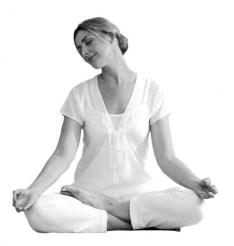

2 Exhale as your head comes back over your left shoulder and round to the front. Keep your jaw relaxed and move in a slow, fluid and meditative rhythm.

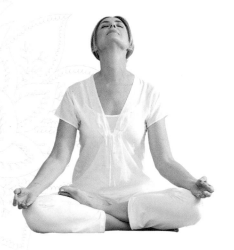

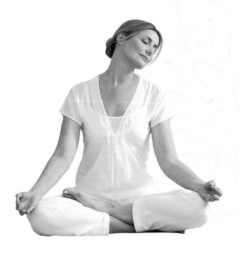

3 After 1–2 minutes come back to the centre and continue the exercise in the opposite direction.

STRETCH POSE

This is a useful exercise for awakening and balancing energy before meditation. I discuss it in the next chapter, as it is also key in raising awareness of your breath and navel centre. See pages 104–105 if you would like to include it in your energy-awakening routine. This powerful exercise fortifies and tones the abdominal area and balances the energy in the digestive and reproductive systems, so you will feel cleansed and strengthened. It also nourishes the navel centre, where the body's 72,000 nadis come together in your centre of gravity and seat of personal power. Stretch Pose is challenging but rewarding – trust that your stamina and confidence will increase. If you feel lacking in motivation with your practice, this is an excellent preparation exercise.

Poses for Meditation and Relaxation

Think of a time when your body was deeply relaxed – perhaps you were on holiday, lying in the sun after a swim. Experiencing such states is essential for physical and mental well-being, yet deep relaxation is often difficult to achieve because our inner emotional dialogue drains our energy. Obsessive negative thoughts and self-destructive emotions such as anger, anxiety and despair directly affect the flow of prana within the body.

To achieve a relaxed and balanced state, you must have a connection between body, mind and soul. Kundalini meditation can help to penetrate the "mask" of your personality, composed of unconscious patterns of being and acting. Making time to meditate and relax each day will guide you into a place where you are able to cope far more easily with life's challenges.

Many energetic and biochemical changes occur after practising Kundalini exercises and meditations, so it is important to give the body and mind time to relax and assimilate the effects. Deep relaxation will improve your capacity to meditate and meditation will teach you to relax. Do not be alarmed if you experience physical discomfort and tension when you practise relaxing, as this is all part of the journey to increasing your awareness.

The simple poses on the next pages are good to experience after the exercises on pages 74–83, during or after the meditations in Chapter 6 or whenever you have a few minutes to spare. Taking time to relax every day can help you to break the stress cycle and let go of negative patterns. As you increase your capacity to meditate, you will become more conscious of how to relax. And this ability to relax will be reflected in your approach to daily life.

OPPOSITE This 12th-century Jain sculpture from Gujarat shows a spiritual seeker who has achieved enlightenment. He is in the Full Lotus pose, with his hands in Dhyana Mudra (the meditation mudra).

PRANA, NADIS AND THE CHAKRAS

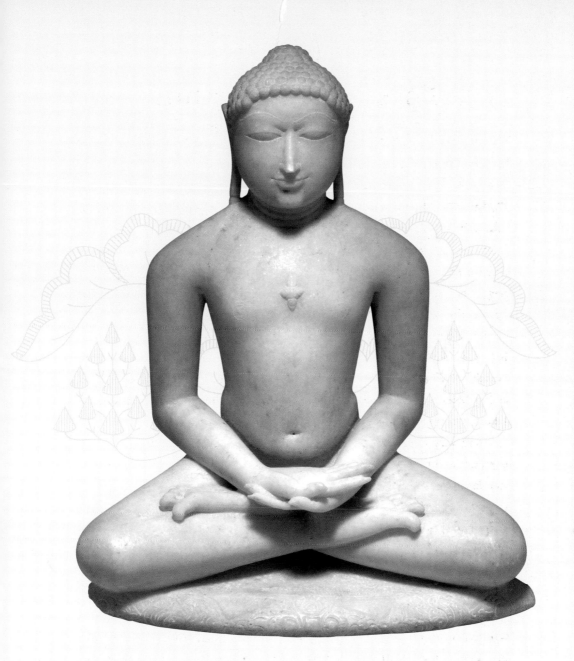

"You should sit in meditation for 20 minutes every day — unless you're too busy; then you should sit for an hour."

Zen saying

Half Lotus

This pose is suitable for people who are unable to get into the Full Lotus position or who find it uncomfortable. With practice this pose is very relaxing and stabilizing. It is effective in Kundalini meditation, providing a firm base for the body and the base chakra.

1 Sit cross-legged, then lift one foot and place it on the opposite thigh. Bring it as high as is comfortable until your foot turns out and the sole faces upward.

2 Keep your lower spine tilted forward, so that your upper spine remains straight, and relax your shoulders.

3 Close your eyes and focus at the third eye between the eyebrows. Breathe long and deep through your nostrils and allow yourself to go into deep relaxation.

Easy Pose

An alternative sitting pose to the Half Lotus is Easy Pose (Sukasana), which also stimulates the base chakra. Great for beginners, this pose is easier on the knees than Lotus Pose and requires less flexibility. If you are sitting for long periods, place a cushion under your bottom to raise your hips higher than your knees.

1 Cross your legs, keeping them relaxed toward the ground. Both feet remain on the ground. Keep your lower back tilted slightly forward so that your upper back remains straight.

2 Close your eyes and focus at the third eye between the eyebrows. Breathe long and deep through your nostrils and allow yourself to go into deep relaxation.

ROCK POSE

This sitting pose, also known as Vajrasana, is a great aid for the digestion. Try it after a meal. If you are uncomfortable sitting on your heels, place a cushion under your bottom.

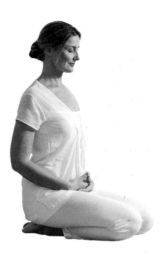

1 Sit on your heels. Keeping your spine straight, relax your hands in your lap or rest them on your thighs.

2 Breathe long and deep through your nostrils, and relax.

BABY POSE

This pose is similar to the position we take as babies in the womb, hence the name. It stimulates the pituitary gland, and helps you to relax completely. If you have low or high blood pressure, or become dizzy, place a mat under your head or rest your head in your hands.

1 Sit on your heels and rest your forehead on the ground. Rest your arms along the sides of your body with your palms facing upward.

2 Close your eyes and focus at the third eye between the eyebrows. Breathe long and deep through your nostrils, relaxing in the pose for at least 3 minutes.

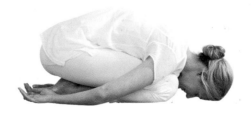

Gurpranam Pose

As well as being relaxing, this variation of Baby Pose brings you an all-knowing, intuitive wisdom. If you are looking for answers, meditate in this position as you breathe long and deep through your nostrils.

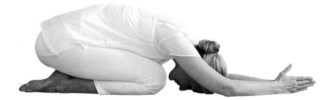

1 Sit on your heels and bring your forehead to the ground, stretching both arms out in front of your head with your palms together.

2 Close your eyes and focus at the third eye between your eyebrows. Breathe long and deep through your nostrils. Observe your breath and surrender to whatever thoughts and feelings come. Let go!

Corpse Pose

Corpse Pose (Shavasana) is the best position for deep relaxation and one of the easiest to fall asleep in! If it helps you to relax, play some calm music as you practise this pose.

1 Lie on your back with your arms at your sides and your palms facing upward. Relax your legs and uncross your ankles. If you feel pressure on your lower back, place a cushion or a blanket under your knees.

2 Tuck your chin in toward your collar bones to lengthen your neck.

3 Close your eyes and breathe long and deep through your nostrils, letting go and releasing every part of your body.

LETTING GO OF TENSION

The breath (see Chapter 4) is a good indicator of how stressed you are feeling – simply by changing the way you breathe, you can bring your body and mind back into energetic balance. If there are situations where you feel you can't slow down, and the stressful experience cannot be changed, try going deeper into your breath or silently chanting the mantra SAT NAM (see page 119) to help to minimize your body's reaction.

1 If you wear glasses or contact lenses, remove them to relax your eyes. Put on some beautiful, inspiring music. Cover yourself with a blanket or a shawl as you relax in any of the poses on pages 86–8.

2 Ask yourself where you feel tension and how your breath is flowing. Feel your body consciously letting go as you close your eyes and relax your lips, tongue, jaw and forehead.

3 Allow your mind to follow the breath and mentally scan your body, from your feet upward. If your mind wanders, bring your awareness back to the breath. Imagine light and energy (prana) coming into your body with each inhalation and feel all the tension and stress leaving your body on each exhalation. If your mind still wanders, try mentally vibrating the mantra SA TA NA MA (see pages 130–31) as you inhale and exhale.

4 Relax in your innermost self for at least 5 minutes and allow your body to absorb the changes and the healing. If you fall asleep, even better, as this will be a very different sleep to any sleep you have experienced before!

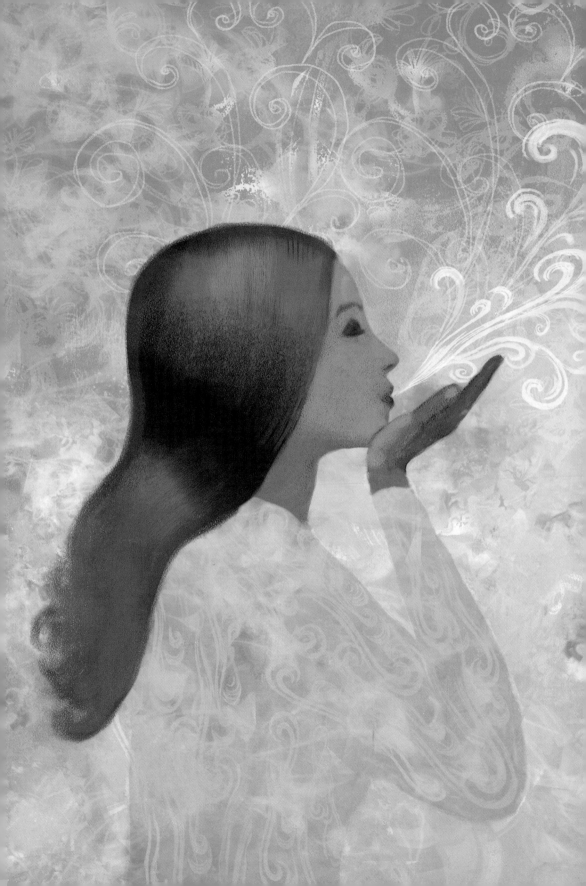

CHAPTER 4

The Power of Breath

Breath is our life-force and one of the most important ways
in which we can work with Kundalini energy. This chapter
provides exercises to help you to perfect your breathing.

"For breath is life, and if you breathe well you will live long on earth."

Sanskrit saying

Kundalini and the Breath

One of the main problems facing us in our world today is stress, and we are all noticing that it is increasing rather than decreasing. Luckily, the quickest and most effective way to cope with stress is very simple: just stop and observe how you are breathing!

Breath is our life-force. Just as we need food and water to sustain us, most importantly we need breath to live. If we can harness the power of our breathing, we can release stress and disease from the body.

Our breath carries prana, the same energy that gives life to all physical matter. If we consciously control our breathing, we can direct this energy in a positive way, to change our physical and psychological health. One of the first things I look at when teaching Kundalini meditation is how people breathe; it reveals a lot about their thoughts and emotional state. People who are anxious and fearful usually breathe in a very shallow, rapid way, from the upper chest rather than using the diaphragm, while those who have a deeper and slower breathing pattern are usually more calm, patient and centred.

The science of yogic breathing is known as pranayama (prana = life-force; pran = first unit; ayam = expansion). Through different breathing techniques we can learn to control the movement of prana and expand our life-force beyond what we thought was possible.

When I first discovered Kundalini yoga I thought I had a deep understanding of how breath works because of my background as a singer, but it wasn't until I explored and experienced Kundalini breathing meditations that I realized I had previously only just touched the surface of what was possible!

Most of us have forgotten how to breathe correctly. We breathe with an irregular rhythm and use only a fraction of our lung capacity. When our inhalation and exhalation are shallow and without rhythm, we feel stressed-out and lacking in vitality, and we don't have sufficient energy to awaken

Kundalini. Before you begin the exercises in this chapter, remind your body of its natural breathing pattern. Sit quietly and observe your breathing: do you breathe from the stomach or from your chest? It's just as important to expel the air fully from your lungs as it is to fill them, so check that you are breathing from the diaphragm.

Exploring your breath through Kundalini meditation will open you to new ways of being. Techniques that look at regulating rhythm, depth and speed of breathing will help you to cope with your different states of emotion and health. When we begin to recognize that the breath is much more than respiration and allow ourselves to experience it as prana moving through us, we can enjoy a new, expanded awareness of our physical, mental and emotional well-being.

BREATHE YOUR STRESS AWAY

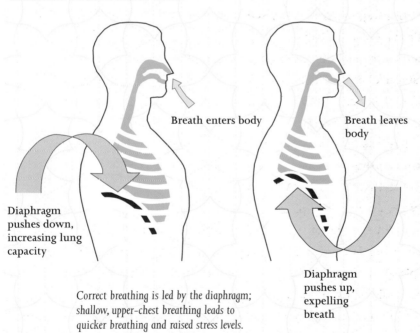

Breath enters body

Breath leaves body

Diaphragm pushes down, increasing lung capacity

Diaphragm pushes up, expelling breath

Correct breathing is led by the diaphragm; shallow, upper-chest breathing leads to quicker breathing and raised stress levels.

The Importance of Pranayama

Pranayama is the art of controlling your breath. Once you are able to control the rhythm of your breathing you can build concentration and positively influence your autonomic nervous system (the involuntary nervous system responsible for bodily responses such as heart rate, perspiration and digestion). A balanced rhythm of breathing involves a good ratio between time spent on inhalation, retention of breath and exhalation; some experts state this to be 1:4:2.

The breathing meditations in this chapter will help you to become much more sensitive to the way prana moves through your subtle body. Consciously choosing to breathe in a deeper, slower and more expansive way will maximize your pranic energy.

The practise of pranayama plays a fundamental role in balancing prana energy with apana energy (see page 66) and in awakening Kundalini. Conscious pranayama can direct and circulate the vital current of prana through the nadis, especially through the major channels known as the ida and pingala (see page 68) and down to the base of the spine where Kundalini energy lies coiled, ready for awakening.

Through breath suspension and the application of body locks (see pages 70–72), apana ascends from the lower chakras to meet prana. When the two energies unite at the solar plexus chakra, a powerful psychic heat is generated that raises Kundalini energy through the chakras (see page 69).

Understanding pranayama is key to understanding Kundalini meditation. It was on these breath techniques that the Tantras placed the most emphasis.

Choose a comfortable position, such as the Half Lotus, in which to practise the breathing exercises. To gain maximum benefit from the exercises, keep your spine straight, your diaphragm open and your head aligned with your body.

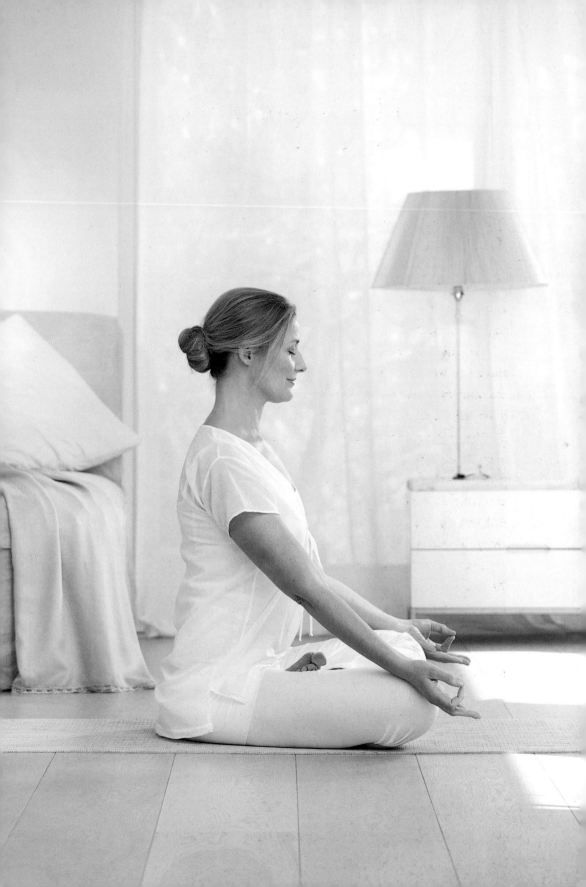

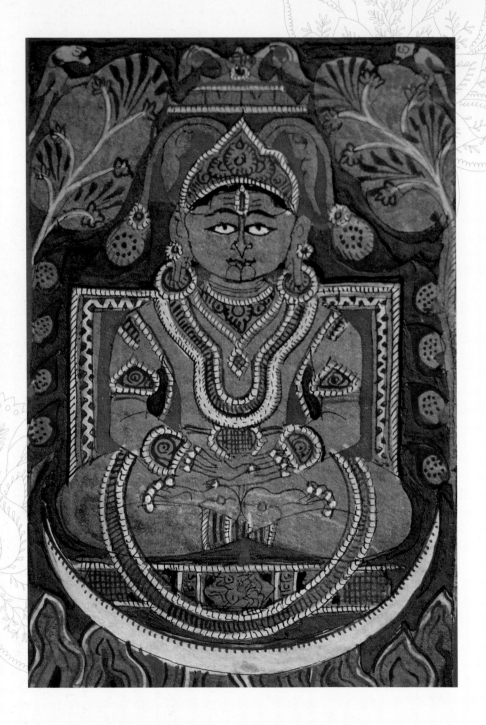

THE POWER OF BREATH

ONE-MINUTE BREATH

This exercise introduces the idea of breath suspension (see pages 100–101), and encourages a deep, expanded breathing pattern. If you are not used to breathing like this, don't be surprised if it feels a little challenging at first!

1 Sit cross-legged with your hands relaxed on your knees in Gyan Mudra (see page 121). If you wish to monitor your breath using a timer you can open your eyes slightly; otherwise, close your eyes and count mentally.

2 Allow the breath to be long, slow and deep into the abdomen as you inhale for 20 seconds. Your abdomen should expand fully and you should feel your chest rising as you receive the inhalation.

3 As you suspend the inhalation for 20 seconds, bring your attention to your upper ribs and your sternum. Gently lift your ribcage as you relax your face and shoulders. Allow your stomach to expand and soften, as you pull your chin in slightly. Feel yourself entering a still, calm place. (If you feel like exhaling before you have suspended the in-breath, try inhaling a little more so that you can extend the time without any stress.)

4 Exhale slowly for 20 seconds, allowing your chest to deflate.

5 Draw your navel in toward your spine. Completely empty your lungs, relaxing your shoulders, face and ribcage.

CAUTION: Beginners should reduce the times to 10 seconds for each inhalation or exhalation and then gradually build to 20 seconds. If you experience a dizzy or faint feeling when holding your breath, reduce the time even further.

OPPOSITE This 15th–16th century Gujarati painting depicts a Jain tirthankara, or one who has achieved enlightenment through meditation and become a role model for other spiritual voyagers.

Developing Breath Awareness

The quality and quantity of your breath, and the way it circulates around your body, all create a strong foundation for an energetic and creative life. Your breath is a good indicator of how much energy you are running on and how much you have in reserve to deal with the stressful situations that inevitably arise in life.

Stress creates the shallow, upper-chest, erratic breathing that is known as clavicular breathing. This breathing pattern eventually leads to muscular tension and affects the nervous system, causing stress. If severe, it becomes hyperventilation, inducing a panic attack.

Correct, diaphragmatic breathing (see box, page 93) will help you to release deep emotional trauma and tension. When we expand our lungs fully, breathe slowly and regularly and allow the flow of prana to circulate through the body, vitality and sensitivity increase. This makes us feel physically stronger and emotionally more secure.

Our capacity for creative expression is also affected by the way in which we breathe. The breath and sound are joined in an intimate relationship. Shortly after we leave the womb, we take our first breath to express our first sound. This signifies that we are alive! Through the ages, spiritual masters and sages have believed that in order to live up to our potential and command our own destiny, we must develop our way of breathing and be conscious of the words we speak and think.

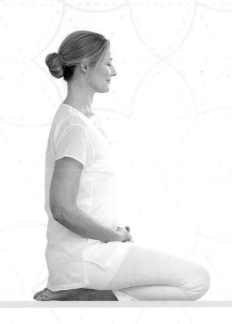

Visualization

One of the most effective ways to develop awareness of your breath is to meditate on it. Take time out to really experience your breath – to listen to it, observe it and become one with it. Give yourself the breath of life!

1 As you sit on your heels with your hands in your lap, close your eyes and roll them in and up toward your third eye.

2 Take a long, slow, deep breath through your nostrils and allow your navel to expand outward.

3 Visualize the prana (subtle life-force) entering your body as a light, cleansing, rejuvenating energy. Feel appreciation and gratitude for this breath.

4 Exhale completely through the nostrils and pull your navel in toward your spine. Visualize apana (eliminating energy) leaving your body. Release all the stale, stagnant energy that is no longer serving you.

5 Let go of any fears or doubts and welcome each new breath!

DEVELOPING BREATH AWARENESS

BREATH SUSPENSION

Breath suspension on an inhalation or exhalation will give you a deeper awareness of prana (life-force) and apana (eliminating energy). It is important to master the suspension of the in-breath and the out-breath, to avoid causing unnecessary tension in your body. If you use the correct technique, described below, you will feel the muscles of your ribs, diaphragm and abdomen relax as you suspend your breath. By training your subconscious mind through repetition of this exercise, you will create a muscular memory so that your body knows what to do without you having to direct your breath consciously. Try this exercise lying down to give you a better sense of which areas in the body need to be relaxed.

1 Inhale deeply through the nostrils and suspend your breath, bringing your attention to your upper ribs and collar bone.

2 Gently lift your upper ribs and feel them suspended in place. As you do this, relax your shoulders, throat and face.

3 Pull in your chin slightly. If you feel the desire to exhale, inhale a little more air. In this moment, allow yourself to experience a sense of profound calm and stillness.

THE BENEFITS OF BREATH SUSPENSION
Breath suspension allows oxygen to penetrate deeply throughout your body. As you practise the technique, you will begin to balance your body's sympathetic and parasympathetic nervous systems and regulate your blood pressure.
You will also boost your concentration and decision-making abilities. With regular practice, you will begin to experience deep stillness and a new way of being – it is in this place that Kundalini energy begins to flow. Over time you will develop a more meditative mind, becoming calmer, happier and more connected to life.

4 Exhale fully and draw your navel in toward your spine.

5 As you suspend your breath, slightly lift your lower chest and diaphragm and allow your upper ribs to relax and come together. As you do this, try not to collapse your spine and ribcage together, as that would disrupt the motion of your diaphragm.

6 Gently pull your chin in and enter into a space of stillness and calm.

7 If you feel yourself struggling for a new breath, consciously exhale a little more air out of your lungs.

BREATH-SUSPENSION TIPS

- Stop if you feel dizzy or disoriented when suspending your breath, as this is not the objective.

- Begin again if you feel you are locking, stiffening or tightening muscles on the suspension of breath.

- Be patient and find a pace that works for you. It takes time to integrate new habits and pushing yourself will only create frustration.

- If levels of carbon dioxide in your blood are too high, your brain will prompt you to inhale. Try exhaling as much air as possible as this will remove carbon dioxide from your blood and help you to suspend inhalation for longer and with more ease.

- Remember that the aim with all breath-suspension techniques is *gradually* to transform your nervous system, emotions and metabolic rate. Begin slowly.

- Observe your mind and body on each breath suspension and explore going deeper, to create that internal place of peace.

The Navel Centre

To understand meditation and the nature of consciousness, it helps to have a clear understanding of the navel centre – the solar plexus (manipura) chakra. This very powerful chakra is a centre for energy transformation in the body. The navel centre or solar plexus chakra is not to be confused with the belly button (umbilicus), although they are related. Some teachers say that the navel centre is located in approximately the same place as the belly button, on the lower spine, while others believe it to be sited 2–3in (5–7.5cm) lower.

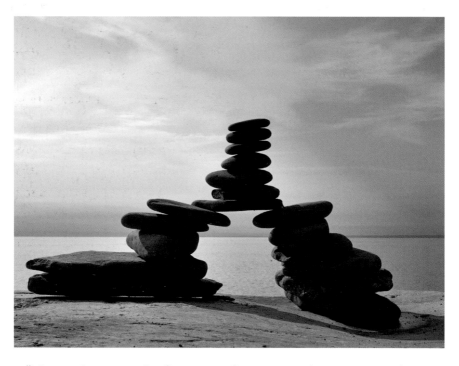

"The navel centre is the first point of awareness when you are exploring balance, strength and movement."

THE POWER OF BREATH

Breathing into the Navel Centre

The navel centre or the solar plexus chakra is the first point of awareness when you are exploring balance, strength and movement in the disciplines of martial arts and yoga. All the body's 72,000 nadi channels meet at this point, and it is through the navel centre that we can harness much energy.

Meditation on the breath at the navel centre is the starting point for awareness of prana. When we are breathing correctly and naturally, the navel moves out on the inhalation, and in and up toward the spine on the exhalation. Most people breathe in the opposite way – that is, they pull the stomach in on the inhalation, which creates less space for the breath in the lungs.

When you are practising this exercise, it is preferable to wear loose clothing, so as not to restrict movement in your diaphragm.

1 Lie down and relax your shoulders. Close your eyes and place your hands over your navel centre, approximately 2–3in (5–7.5cm) below your belly button. Breathe naturally through your nose and check that your navel is moving correctly: out on the in-breath and in and up on the out-breath.

2 If you feel that the connection between your breath and your navel seems weak, practise Stretch Pose (see pages 104–105). This is one of the most effective ways to locate the pulse of the navel centre and build energy there.

STRETCH POSE

This powerful exercise builds awareness of prana and the functioning of your navel centre. It is also one of the key practices to awaken energy in preparation for meditation (see pages 73–83). Even if you can only hold the position for a few seconds, it will feel rewarding and ignite confidence!

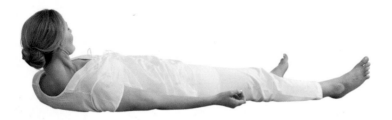

1   Lie on your back, with your arms relaxed by your side, and stretch out your spine. Tilt your pelvis slightly forward, so as to take any pressure off your lower back. Raise your head to look at your feet.

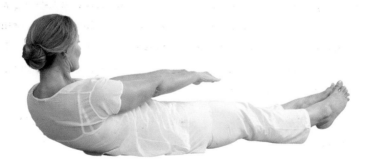

2   Raise your upper back and legs 6in (15cm) off the ground, stretching out your arms above your legs. (If you have lower back problems, place your hands under your buttocks.)

3 Tuck your chin into your chest and look toward your big toes. Try to hold this position for 1–2 minutes while you do a Breath of Fire (see page 107) to bring out the navel pulse – a rapid and equal inhalation and exhalation through the nostrils coordinated with the navel. If you are a beginner, start slowly and feel the pulse at the navel as you breathe.

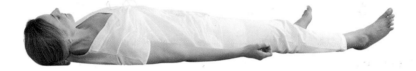

4 When you have finished, relax into Corpse Pose (see page 88).

5 Place the tips of two fingers on top of your belly button. Press firmly toward your spine and you will find a point that beats rhythmically and strongly. If you feel this beat exactly in your navel centre (about 2–3in/ 5-7.5cm below the belly button), then it usually means the energy at this point is balanced. If you feel the beat off-centre, then keep practising Stretch Pose to bring your navel centre back into alignment.

CAUTION: Do not practise Stretch Pose if you are pregnant or menstruating heavily. Try to avoid eating for three hours beforehand.

Exercises to Master Breath

Here are a few suggestions for other breathing techniques that will help you to master your breath and develop an awareness of prana and apana. All these exercises will help you to control your emotions and develop a meditative mind. With practice, you will become calmer, healthier and happier.

LONG, DEEP BREATHING

By taking deep yogic breaths and breathing into your belly, diaphragm and upper lungs, you have the potential to expand your lungs to several times their normal size. Each part of the breath-expansion process is distinct and when all three areas are expanded, you have a complete long, deep breath. This breathing also helps to:

- increase the flow of prana;

- stimulate endorphins, the chemicals that fight depression;

- stimulate the pituitary gland, increasing your intuition;

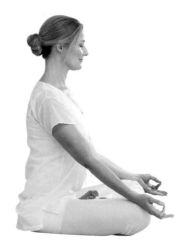

- break your subconscious habits of fear and insecurity;

- pump spinal fluid to the brain, giving you energy and endurance;

- regulate the body's pH (acid–alkaline) balance, helping your metabolic processes;

- relax the body, easing stress.

1 Sitting in Half Lotus or Easy Pose (see page 86) with hands in Gyan Mudra (see page 121) on your knees, close your eyes and focus at the third eye.

2 Stretch tall through your spine and relax your shoulders.

3 Feel the breath flow as you slowly inhale through your nostrils, expanding your abdomen and chest and gently lifting your upper ribs and collar bones.

4 As you exhale through your nostrils, reverse the process. Relax your collar bones, empty your chest and pull your abdomen in and up as the navel pulls back toward the spine – emptying any last drop of air from the lungs.

BREATH OF FIRE

This powerful, energizing breath will cleanse your blood and increase the flow of oxygen to your brain. It will strengthen your navel centre and your nervous and immune systems, bringing you back into balance. After practising this for just 1–2 minutes, you will feel rejuvenated and revitalized!

1 Sitting in Half Lotus or Easy Pose (see page 86) with hands in Gyan Mudra (see page 121) on your knees, close your eyes and focus at the third eye.

2 Start to inhale and exhale through your nostrils with your mouth closed. This is a powerful, rapid breath (aim for 2–3 breaths per second) powered from the navel, with no pause between the inhalation and the exhalation.

3 As you exhale, powerfully pull your navel and abdomen in toward your spine. When you inhale, release your navel to allow the breath to inflate the lungs.

4 If you are new to this breath, focus on the exhalation, placing one hand on your navel to feel its movement as you do so. Begin slowly to find your rhythm and the balance between your breath and your navel, feeling the inward pull on the exhale and the release on the inhale.

CAUTION: Do not practise this breath if you are pregnant or menstruating heavily.

Alternate Nostril Breathing

Your nostrils act as entry points to the pranic body and regulate body temperature and energy. Breathing long and deep through the left nostril activates the right side of the brain and your moon energy, which is cooling, calming and mind-expanding. Breathing through the right nostril activates the left side of the brain and your sun energy, which is dynamic, action-oriented and mentally alert. The right nostril (sun energy) links to the positive nadi (pingala) and the left nostril (moon energy) links to the negative nadi (ida). As we breathe, we automatically switch dominant nostril every 90–150 minutes, regulated by the hypothalamus and the pituitary gland.

1 Sit in Half Lotus or Easy Pose (see page 86) with your spine straight and mentally prepare to use your right thumb and index finger to close alternate nostrils. Focus at the third eye (your eyes can be open or closed).

2 Close your right nostril with your thumb and inhale deeply through your left nostril.

3 After a full inhalation, close your left nostril with the index finger and exhale fully through your right nostril.

4 Now inhale deeply through your right nostril, and then close it off with your thumb and exhale fully thought your left nostril.

5 Repeat several times, breathing fully on the inhalation and exhalation.

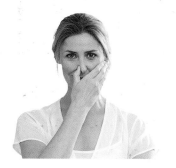 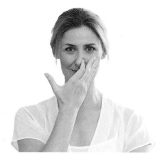

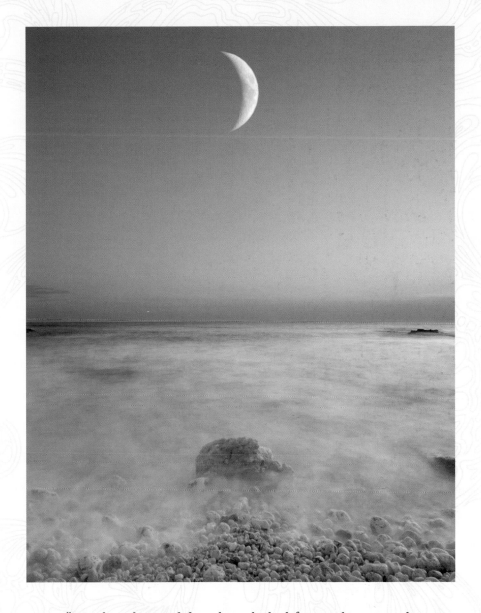

"Breathing long and deep through the left nostril activates the
right side of the brain and your moon energy, which is cooling,
calming and mind-expanding."

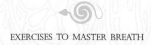

EXERCISES TO MASTER BREATH

CANNON BREATH

This breath cleanses and strengthens your nerves and navel point. It is Breath of Fire (see page 107) through an open mouth. Sitting in Half Lotus or Easy Pose (see page 86) with your hands in Gyan Mudra (see page 121), form an "O" shape with your mouth and focus at the third eye (eyes can be open or closed). Begin a powerful Breath of Fire, feeling the pressure in your cheeks.

WHISTLE BREATH

This exercise combines breathing with sound to circulate your prana and shift your consciousness to a higher level. Through the nervous system, you will stimulate your thyroid and parathyroid glands, and you will feel your lungs expanding.

1 Sitting in Half Lotus or Easy Pose (see page 86) with your hands in Gyan Mudra (see page 121), form an "O" shape with your mouth. Focus at the third eye (your eyes can be open or closed).

2 Inhale through your puckered mouth, making a high-pitched whistle sound.

3 Exhale through your lips.

4 Listen to the sound carried on your breath, going deeper into the sound vibration with each breath.

VARIATION: Try inhaling through your nose and exhaling through your lips as you whistle.

LION BREATH

This dynamic, cleansing breath is great for opening the throat chakra and stimulating the thyroid gland.

1 Sitting in Half Lotus or Easy Pose (see page 86) with your hands in Gyan Mudra (see page 121), open your mouth and extend your tongue as far as possible. Focus at the third eye (your eyes can be open or closed). Breathe powerfully through your mouth.

2 Feel the pressure build in your upper chest and over the root of your tongue.

SITALI BREATH

This cooling breath relaxes and soothes the spine, regulating creative, sexual and digestive energies. It is great if you want to release anger or lower body temperature. Don't worry if you notice a bitter taste on your tongue at first. This means you are detoxing. If you practise regularly, you will feel cleansed and rejuvenated.

1 Sitting in Half Lotus or Easy Pose (see page 86) with your hands in Gyan Mudra (see page 121), focus at the third eye (your eyes can be open or closed). Curl up the sides of your tongue to make a small hole (or bend up its sides as far as you can). Inhale long and deep through this, then exhale through your nostrils as you close your mouth.

VARIATION: Try inhaling and exhaling through your curled tongue.

EXERCISES TO MASTER BREATH

Circular
Breathing

Circular breathing is well known in Tantric practice as a technique to raise sexual energy up the spine through the chakras. It works on the principle of transforming sexual energy into spiritual energy and can be practised on your own or with a partner to enhance your relationship. The energy can be channelled to heal glands and organs and to clear the chakras.

1 Try practising circular breathing lying down at first and then sitting up. Close your eyes and centre yourself at the navel centre (solar plexus chakra). Many teachers believe the navel centre to be about 2–3in (5–7.5cm) below the belly button (see pages 102–103); the exercises in this chapter will help you locate it exactly. Place your thumbs on the navel point and point your fingers down toward the groin area to form a triangle. When you feel emotionally balanced and centred at this point, pranic and sexual energy will flow and Kundalini can awaken. A good way to ignite and balance energy at the navel is to practise Stretch Pose (see pages 104–105) with Breath of Fire (see page 107).

2 As you inhale several long, deep breaths through your nostrils (or take powerful sniffs), feel your navel expand outward and the energy flow down from your navel and up through your spine in the following order:

1 Base of the spine (base chakra)

2 Sex organs (sacral chakra)

3 Navel (solar plexus chakra)

4 Heart (heart chakra)

5 Back of the neck, in line with the throat (throat chakra)

6 Centre of the head, in line with the third eye (third eye chakra)

7 Top of the head (crown chakra)

3 At the end of the inhale squeeze the Root Lock (see page 70), contracting your anus, sex organs and navel. Press your tongue to the roof of your mouth and roll your eyes up, as though you are looking out through the top of your head. Tuck your chin in slightly. Feel the energy at the top of your head as you hold your breath. See the space expanding and enjoy the experience for as long as you like.

4 Exhale, slowly releasing the energy down the front of your body, to the third eye, throat and heart chakras, and so on. Let your breath come naturally. Observe how it carries your energy. With practice you can expand the circle of energy beyond your body, visualizing it expanding with each breath.

CIRCULAR-BREATHING TIPS

- Move energy gently through the breath. Don't try to force it.

- As you breathe, consciously connect the base of your spine with the third eye.

- Synchronizing the breath while feeling and visualizing the energy will help you direct energy up through your spine and back down the front of your body.

- As you hold the inhalation, you could mentally repeat a mantra such as SA TA NA MA (see pages 130–31).

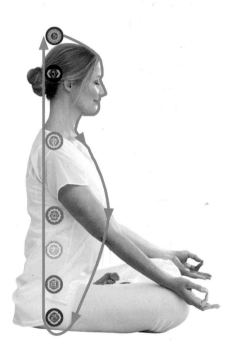

In circular breathing, prana flows down from the navel centre and around all the major chakras.

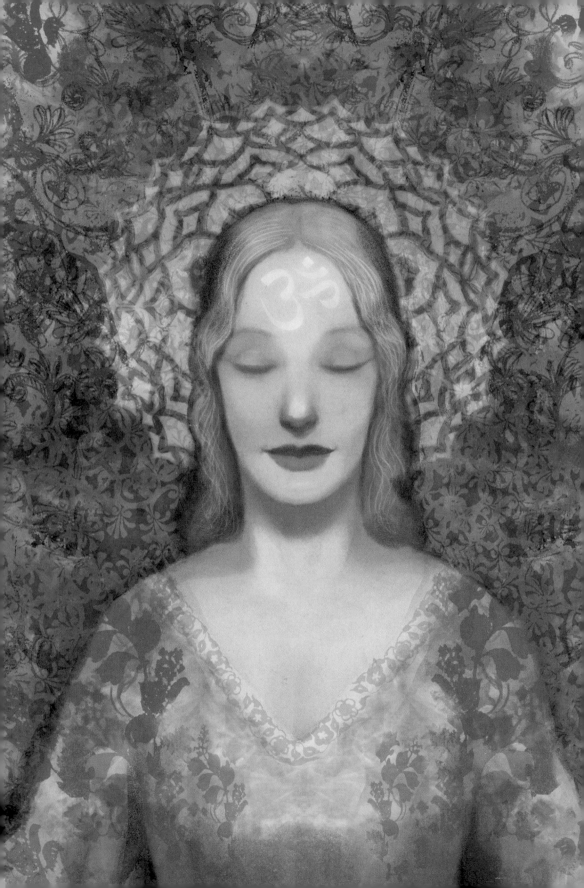

CHAPTER 5

Mantras, Mudras and Yantras

This chapter explores some of the most powerful and spiritually charged tools of Kundalini – mantras (sacred sounds), mudras (hand gestures rich with meaning) and yantras (inspiring sacred diagrams).

EK ONG KAR, SAT NAM, SIRI WAHE GURU
"There is one Creator whose name is Truth.
Great is the ecstasy of that Supreme Wisdom."

Adi Shakti Mantra

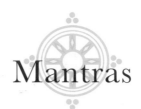

Mantras

Mantras are a powerful component of Kundalini. The term is derived from two Sanskrit words: "manas", or "mind", and "trai", or "to free from". So, "mantra", in its most literal sense, means "to free from the mind".

A mantra consists of one or more syllables (see pages 118–19) that create sound waves. Sound is a form of energy. The sound wave formed by our words determines our feelings and what we project to others. When we vibrate a mantra, we cut through our mental chatter to create inner stillness and focus. The combination of sound, rhythm, tone and meaning clears the mind of ego-driven thoughts that prevent us from experiencing clarity, peace and joy.

Mantras are often in a sacred language, such as Sanskrit. By chanting mantras, we consciously redirect our flow of thoughts, invoking the positive vibration of the syllables. Whether a mantra is for peace, intuition or prosperity, the sound wave leaves no space for other thoughts. It doesn't matter if we don't understand the meaning: the sounds are a formula that elevates consciousness.

Most mantras are chanted in a monotone, although some are sung. It is the repetition of the sound vibration that changes our mental patterns and brain chemistry. Repeatedly chanting a mantra stimulates reflex points on the upper palate that activate the hypothalamus, a gland in the brain, and benefit the whole body. When you chant the mantra meditations in this book, exaggerate the movements with your mouth and tongue to familiarize yourself with the mantra and gain maximum benefit.

Even though I am a trained singer, I found mantras strange at first. However, I let go of my judgment and now enjoy chanting mantras daily. They transport my mind to a place of real peace and are also very effective for opening the chakras, especially the heart and throat chakras. One of my favourite mantras is WAHE GURU (see page 142). It cuts through darkness and negativity, removes the blocks that hold me back, and creates a feeling of gratitude and joy.

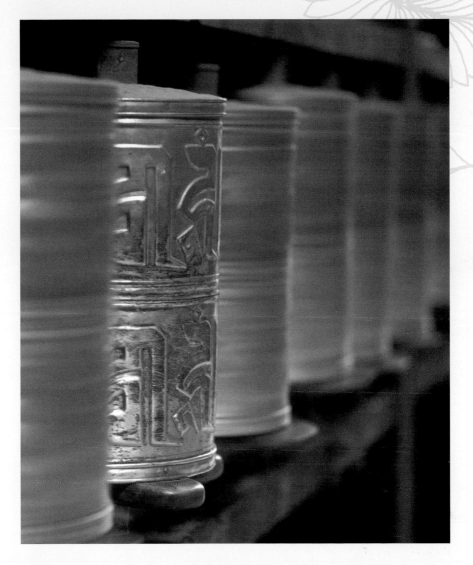

Buddhist prayer wheels, like these at the Jokhang Temple in Lhasa, Tibet, contain thousands of printed mantras that are sent out to the universe with each whirling of a wheel. The Sanskrit mantra OM MANI PADME HUM is traditionally engraved on the exterior of each wheel.

Seed Syllables

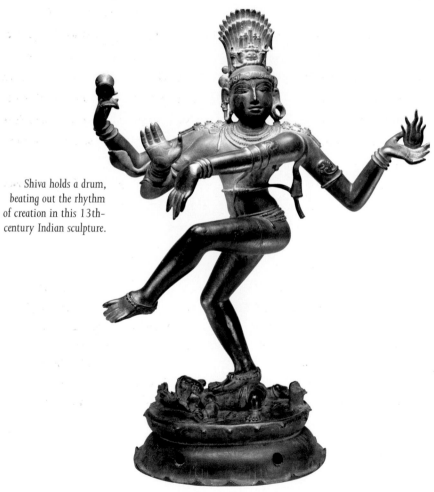

According to ancient texts, all the sounds of the Sanskrit alphabet emerged at Creation, when Shiva danced the world into existence accompanied by the beating of a drum. Sound is powerfully sacred and can help us to awaken to the ultimate reality.

Shiva holds a drum, beating out the rhythm of creation in this 13th-century Indian sculpture.

Seed syllables, or bija, are units of sound in sacred languages such as Sanskrit or Gurmukhi and are often used together, or individually, as mantras. By themselves, seed syllables may not have any literal meaning but they take on great significance within the complete phrase of the mantra.

The most widely used and best-known mantra in Kundalini is SAT NAM, known as the Seed Mantra. SAT means "truth" and NAM means "identity", or "to call on the truth". Chanting these syllables awakens the soul and can rearrange habit patterns in the subconscious mind.

Another well-known seed syllable mantra used in Kundalini is ONG, which by itself cannot be translated literally, although it is regarded as the primal vibration from which all creativity flows (see pages 32–3). It starts many mantras including the Adi Mantra: ONG NAMO, GURU DEV NAMO ("I bow to the creative wisdom, I bow to the divine teacher within"), which traditionally precedes all Kundalini practice and allows us to tune in to the higher self (see pages 58–9). This seed syllable also starts ONG SO HUNG, a heart-opening and empowering mantra that translates as "Creator, I am Thou."

The third main seed mantra in Kundalini is HAR. This stands for prosperity and personal power, as well as the creative aspect of infinity.

ANCIENT SOUNDS

The base chakra, muladhara chakra, is called "the birthplace of all sounds", reflecting the fact that Kundalini lies at this chakra and Kundalini is the origin of original, cosmic sound. According to ancient Hindu texts there are four types of sound. Vaikhari is audible sound; madhyama is the point between audible sound and inner vibration; pashyanti is sound heard only by those who are spiritually awakened; and para (derived from the Sanskrit word for "transcendental") is sound beyond vibration or wavelength – it is the potential for sound.

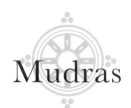

Mudras

L ike mantras, mudras (hand gestures) are an important aspect of Kundalini practice and can help you to progress on your meditation journey. Mudras are found in Hindu, Buddhist, Sikh and other traditions and often feature in religious artwork, such as statues and wall paintings of the Buddha, other deities and the Sikh Gurus. By showing these figures with their hands in particular positions, key messages about the meaning of the artwork could be conveyed directly to the faithful.

In your Kundalini practice, mudras can awaken energies to expand your awareness. Mudras are used in conjunction with pranayama, boosting the flow of prana and intensifying concentration.

Poses for practising mudras

The Half Lotus and Easy Pose (see page 86) are both comfortable siting postures and are excellent for practising mudras. If you have trouble sitting, place a cushion under your buttocks to raise your hips above your knees. At the same time, apply a gentle Neck Lock (see page 72). Rock Pose (see page 87) is also a comfortable position for practising mudras – and has the added benefit of helping the digestion!

The Full Lotus is more difficult to achieve, but it is great for practising mudras as it offers a strong foundation and helps to focus your activated energy. Sit cross-legged with your left foot on your right thigh and your right foot on your left thigh. Keep your knees on the ground, and your spine straight. If this posture doesn't come easily, don't force it. As you work through your session, alternate the top and bottom legs.

Using Mudras in Kundalini

A variety of powerful mudras feature in Kundalini. Choose a mudra that resonates with the problem or situation you are trying to address.

Gyan Mudra
Join the tip of your index finger to the tip of your thumb. This is a receptive mudra, generating knowledge, wisdom and expansion.

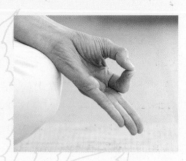

Shuni Mudra
Join the tip of your middle finger to the tip of your thumb to generate patience.

Surya Mudra
Join the tip of your fourth finger to the tip of your thumb to generate vibrant sun energy.

Buddhi Mudra
Join the tip of your little finger to the tip of your thumb to support clear communication.

Prayer Mudra
Press your palms together into the centre of your chest at your heart. Keeping your thumbs straight, press your knuckles into your sternum. To increase pressure in your palms, bring your elbows slightly forward. This mudra neutralizes the positive and negative energies of the left and right brain hemispheres.

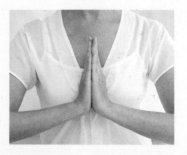

Venus Lock

Interlace your fingers, resting your top thumb on the mound of Venus (the fleshy part between thumb and index finger). Women keep the left thumb on top and men keep the right thumb on top. This mudra channels sexual energy and creates glandular balance.

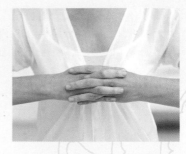

Buddha Mudra

Women place the left hand in the right hand, and men place the right hand in the left hand. Touch your thumb tips and cross your index fingers at right angles near the upper knuckle, to help balance your brain hemispheres and access the neutral, meditative mind.

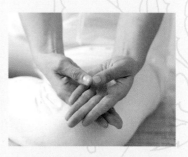

Christ Mudra

"Seal" your ring and little fingers with your thumb, while extending your index and middle fingers, to balance the water and fire elements within your body.

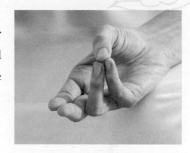

Praying Mantis Mudra

Join all your fingertips at the tip of your thumb, to balance the five elements of the conscious and subconscious mind.

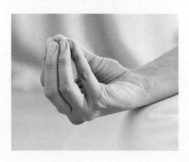

Lotus Mudra

Bring the bases of your hands together, joining your little fingertips and your thumb sides. Imagine you are creating a lotus flower as you open and spread the remaining fingers. Often placed on the heart, throat or the third eye, this mudra balances the five elements of the conscious and subconscious mind.

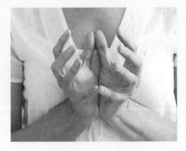

Yoni Mudra

Touch your thumb sides together and bend them back toward your chest, while touching the little fingertips and pointing them forward. Spread out the other three fingers parallel to each other and to the earth. This is a Tantric mudra, balancing male and female energy.

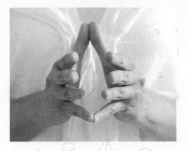

Bear Grip

Hold your left palm facing away from your chest, and your right palm facing toward your chest. Keep your fingers together and curled, creating a firm grip. This mudra stimulates the heart and focuses the mind. It can be practised with a suspended inhalation or exhalation while firmly pulling the finger lock.

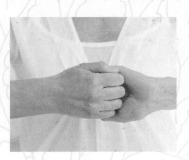

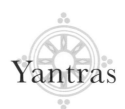

Yantras

In Kundalini practice, illustrations of the chakras are known as yantras. Like mudras, yantras are a visual symbol of the divine, and meditating on them can bring about deeper levels of awareness.

The development of Tantrism, which was so important to Kundalini, also saw a revival of interest in sacred geometry and it was from this discipline that yantras arose. In Tantrism a wide range of visual, aural and gestural symbols (yantras, mantras and mudras) all became an important part of worship, inspiring visualizations and meditations.

The yantra is generally a square that marks sacred space, usually with circles and triangles within, and a central dot, the bindu, that provides a focus for meditation. Yantras are believed to show the essential forms found in the universe – the abstract basis of all matter. The Tantric texts stated that any structure – from a flower to a mountain – has an invisible yantra, its essential subtle form. Human psychology too, can be represented by yantras.

Just as mudras and mantras only become activated by the energy of the person using them, so yantras can become energetically charged as we work with them. In this way the yantra becomes a "power-diagram" that can transform ordinary experience into a rich, spiritual moment of enlightenment. Yantras may seem at one level simple and easy to understand, but this is deceptive. There are multiple layers of spiritual and psychological truth hidden within them, and this is only revealed through meditation and inner vision.

In traditional art, yantras may be engraved, embossed on plates of metal or crystal, or simply traced with vermilion or sandalwood paste. They often incorporate mantras, because in many traditions sound is as important as form. Yantras can always be studied at both a cosmic and a personal level. One of the great principles of Kundalini is the integration of the outer world with the inner world, so every yantra can work at both levels.

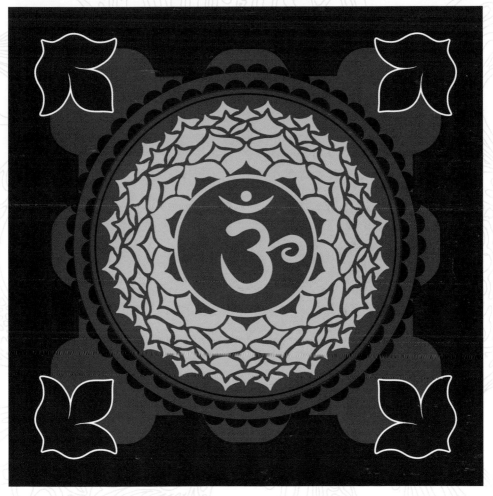

This contemporary yantra representing the crown or sahasrara chakra includes a mass of petals to symbolize the thousand lotus petals traditionally associated with this chakra.

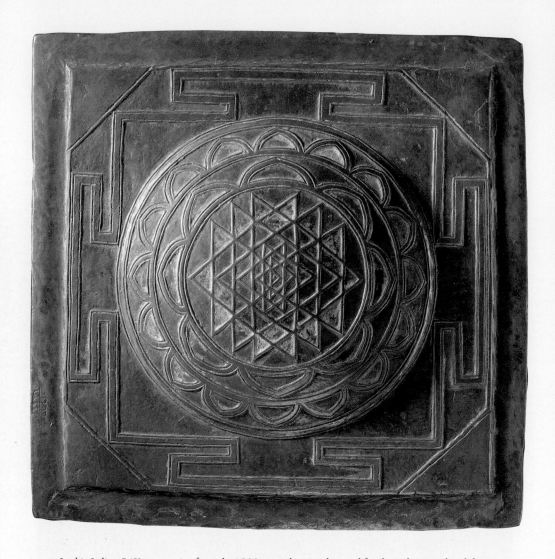

In this Indian Sri Yantra carving from the 1800s, upright triangles stand for the male principle, while downward-pointing triangles represent the female: the whole is a Tantric symbol of unity.

Sri Yantra

One of the most significant yantras is the Sri Yantra or Sri Chakra. This is the Yantra of Creation, also called the Mother of All Yantras because all other yantras derive from it. The Sri Yantra is known in the Hindu, Vedic and Buddhist traditions as the most powerful and mystically beautiful of all yantras. It represents the timeless creative principle of the universe, the continuous unfolding of all realms of creation from the central source. With that in mind, it is used as an object of meditation.

The Sri Yantra is a configuration of nine interlacing triangles centred around the bindu (the central point of the yantra, representing transcendental unity and the source of creation). Five downward-pointing triangles represent Shakti, the female principle, and four upright triangles represent Shiva, the male principle. All the triangles emerge from a central point, standing for the union of male and female, of Shiva and Shakti. Around the chakra image are several concentric circles of lotuses, and the figure is bounded by a square with four sacred doors opening to the four cardinal directions. This yantra symbolizes the journey of Kundalini energy through the chakras that will culminate in the union of Shiva and Shakti at the crown chakra (see pages 28–9).

The Sri Yantra also maps our spiritual journey from material existence to ultimate enlightenment. The spiritual journey is taken as a pilgrimage in which every step is an ascent to the centre, a movement beyond one's limited existence, and every level is nearer to the goal. Each of the circuits of the Sri Yantra, from the outer plane to the central bindu, corresponds with one of the stages of the spiritual journey. Yantras can be powerful tools in your Kundalini practice and there are many different ways you can work with them. For example, meditating on beautiful images of the chakras can be a very effective part of your practice, increasing your awareness of them.

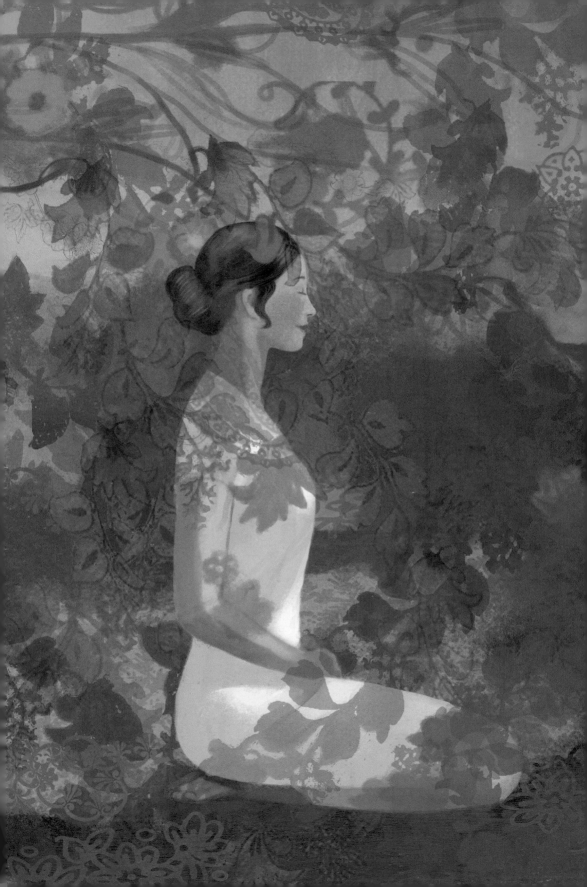

CHAPTER 6

Meditations for Body, Mind and Spirit

In this final chapter I share with you some wonderful
guided Kundalini meditations, each with their own posture,
breath, mantra and mudra. All focus on different aspects of
your life and being.

*"Meditation brings wisdom; lack of meditation leaves ignorance. Know
well what leads you forward and what holds you back, and choose the
path that leads to wisdom."*

Gautama Buddha (c. 563–c. 483 BCE)

Meditation for Emotional Balance and Intuition

This meditation, known as Kirtan Kriya, creates emotional balance and increases intuition. Practising it will bring mental calm and strengthen your sense of self, as well as energizing your aura. It is especially helpful for women and can be used to cope with hormonal imbalances. It is also very good if you are pregnant. I love this meditation as it helps to release a lot of emotions and always brings me back to a place of deep inner calm and connection.

During this meditation you will use a mantra made up of five primal sounds – S, T, N, M, A, in their word form. Chanting these sounds allows you to tap into the continuous cycle of creation:

SA ("saah") – "infinity" in Sanskrit
TA ("taah") – "life"
NA ("naah") – "death"
MA ("maah") – "rebirth"

There is a special mudra associated with each sound of the mantra. Move your fingers through the mudras as you chant the syllables. In each case the tip of the thumb should create a firm pressure as it touches the tip of the other finger.

SA – Thumb and index finger (Gyan Mudra – for knowledge)
TA – Thumb and middle finger (Shuni Mudra – for patience)
NA – Thumb and fourth finger (Surya Mudra – for vitality)
MA – Thumb and little finger (Buddhi Mudra – for communication)

1   Sit in Half Lotus or Easy Pose (see page 86) and apply a light Neck Lock (see page 72). Keep your arms straight, with hands in Gyan Mudra (see page 121).

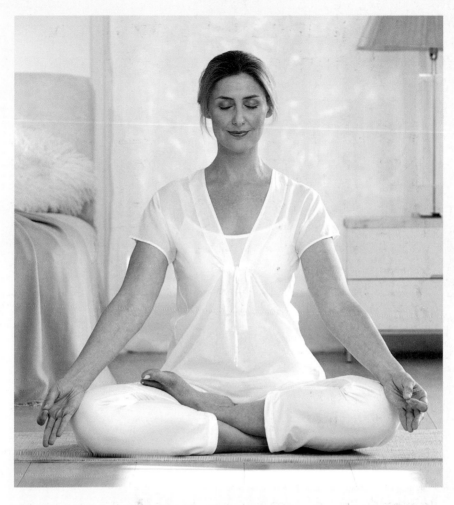

2 Close your eyes and focus at the third eye point.

3 Chant the mantra in three different voices for different lengths of time: normal (out loud) – 5 minutes; whispered – 5 minutes; inward (silent) – 10 minutes. As you work through the mantra syllables, adopt the correct mudras.

4 After the inward chant, return to the whispered voice for 5 minutes and finish chanting with the normal voice (out loud) for 5 minutes. (This meditation takes a total of 30 minutes, but the times can be reduced as long as you maintain the time ratio between the different voices.)

Meditation to Break Habits and Heal Addictions

Most of us have experienced an addiction of some kind. If we are not addicted to emails, texting, shopping, smoking, drugs, food, alcohol, sex or television, then we are addicted to fear of failure or rejection. All these forms of addiction can lead to insecure, neurotic patterns of behaviour.

An imbalance in the pineal area affects other brain glands, and can create unhealthy habits, fears or addictions. In this meditation, the pressure of your thumbs on your skull activates the central brain area, triggering the pineal gland. If the pineal area is balanced, your mind and body will be in harmony and you will fly free. This meditation is especially effective for those in rehabilitation for drug dependence, mental illness or phobic conditions. I gave this meditation to a student who was desperate to give up smoking. He committed to it for 120 days and now no longer smokes!

1 Sit in Half Lotus or Easy Pose (see page 86) with a light Neck Lock (see page 72). Close your eyes and focus at the third eye.

2 Make fists with your hands and extend your thumbs, pressing them firmly on your temples. Clench your back molars, keeping your mouth closed.

3 Silently vibrate the mantra SA TA NA MA ("saah, taah, naah, maah"), firmly squeezing your back molars together on each sound, then releasing the pressure. You should be able to feel the muscles moving under your thumbs as you squeeze your back teeth.

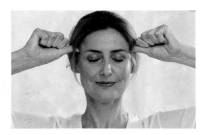

4 Choose one addiction or habit and practise daily for up to 31 minutes. After 40 days you will really notice a shift.

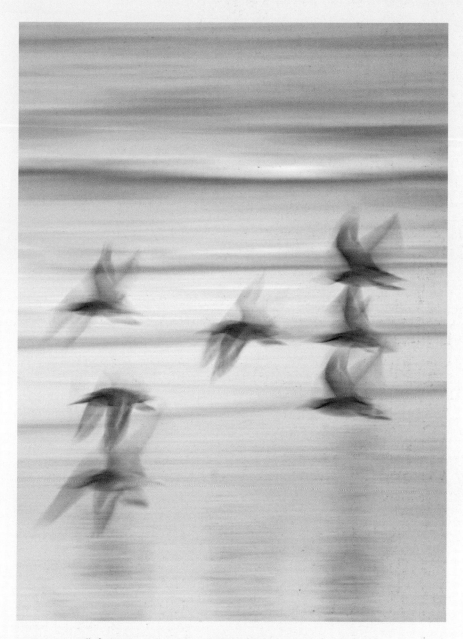

"If the pineal area is balanced, your mind and body

will be in harmony and you will fly free."

Meditation to Release Anger

Anger is a powerful emotion that can be transformed into love, peace and forgiveness. This meditation will release your anger and calm your mind, bringing you back to a state of real peace and wisdom. I enjoy this meditation as it is very invigorating as well as effective in releasing anger.

1 Sit straight in Half Lotus or Easy Pose (see page 86) with your eyes either open or closed. Apply a light Neck Lock (see page 72).

2 Make tight fists with your hands in front of your solar plexus.

3 Create a space between each fist and then powerfully open your forearms, keeping your elbows parallel to the ground.

4 As your fists come back, cross your forearms at the chest area. Powerfully chant the mantra HAR, which denotes the creative aspect of infinity. Pull your navel in as you chant "HAR!", and roll the "R", striking your tongue on the roof of your mouth. This action stimulates the hypothalamus, shifting you into the neutral, meditative mind.

5 Continue for 5–7 minutes, keeping the movement rhythmic, forceful and strong. Feel your whole body vibrating with the sound and movement. See yourself breaking the chains of anger and frustration, clearing those emotions that restrict you. Put all your energy into this meditation. Now is your chance to let go of any anger that you have been holding onto!

6 To finish, inhale deeply and squeeze your fists firmly in front of your chest. Hold for a few seconds and then exhale. Repeat this two more times, making your fists even tighter. Relax.

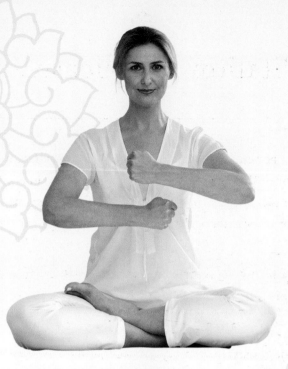

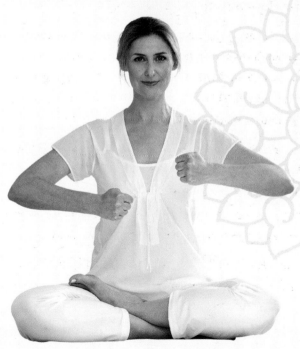

Meditation for Healing

This beautiful, healing mantra meditation (known as the Siri Gaitri Mantra) will connect you to the cycle of infinite energy and open you to healing and awareness. It is wonderful to chant in a group, when you can really feel its vibration. The eight sounds – RA MA DA SA, SA SAY SO HUNG – stimulate Kundalini energy and activate the neutral mind. The meditation has been useful for some students of mine who were anxious before medical procedures.

RA ("raah") denotes the sun. It energizes and purifies.
MA ("maah") denotes the moon. It cools and nurtures.
DA ("daah") denotes the Earth. It grounds you.
SA ("saah") denotes infinity.
SAY SO HUNG denotes your experience of merging with the infinite.

1 Sit in Half Lotus or Easy Pose (see page 86) with a light Neck Lock (see page 72) and close your eyes. Relax your elbows against your ribs and extend your forearms out from your body. Keep your palms flat and facing up, your wrists slightly pulled back and your fingers together, with your thumbs spread.

2 Chant one complete cycle of the mantra RA MA DA SA, SA SAY SO HUNG, pulling your navel point in on SO and HUNG. As you chant this mantra from the heart, feel yourself connecting to each sound, allowing the vibration to resonate in your mouth and sinuses. Continue for up to 11 minutes.

3 To finish, inhale and hold your breath, offering a healing prayer to someone who needs healing (perhaps to yourself). See this person healthy, happy and strong. You can send as many prayers for healing as you like.

4 Afterwards, shake out your arms and sit in silence for a few minutes.

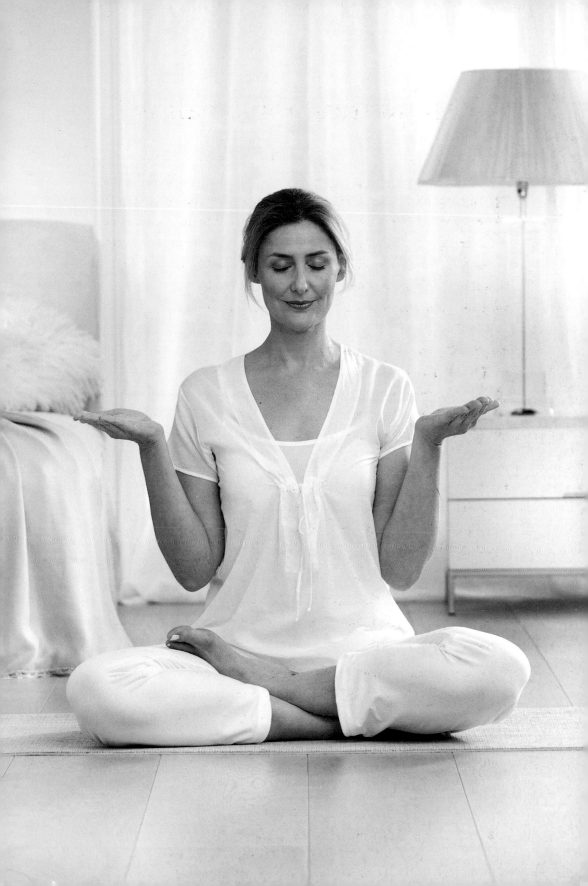

Meditation to Boost the Immune System

This is a deeply cleansing meditation that boosts your immune system. It clears out viruses and bacteria, leaving your whole body rejuvenated. It removes blocks caused by destructive emotions, such as anger, blame and guilt, from your central nervous and endocrine systems. This meditation also stimulates and re-balances the right hemisphere of the brain. This part of the brain can store negative emotions, causing depression and a weakened immune system.

Don't be surprised if the process releases mixed emotions as your body's glands adjust. Keep breathing and trust that you will reach a place where you feel positive, light and energized. I practise this meditation whenever I am feeling run down from a heavy work schedule, and immediately feel protected and revitalized.

1 Sit in Half Lotus or Easy Pose (see page 86) with a light Neck Lock (see page 72).

2 Bend your left arm and raise your hand to shoulder level with your palm facing forward. Join the tip of your thumb with the tip of your fourth finger (Surya Mudra, see page 121). Try to keep this mudra in your left hand at shoulder level throughout the meditation.

3 Create a fist with your right hand, extending your index finger to close off your right nostril. Close your eyes and focus on the third eye.

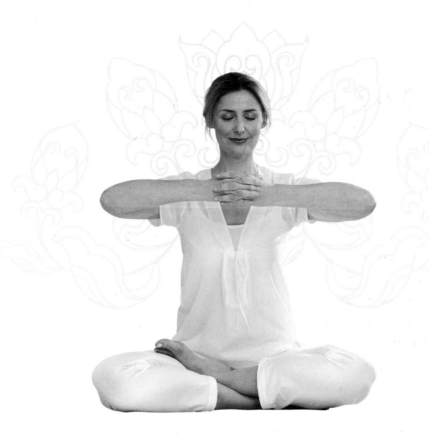

4 Begin a powerful and steady Breath of Fire (see page 107) through your left nostril.

5 Pulse your navel rhythmically as you breathe. Imagine you are creating a drum beat with your navel point. Continue for 3–5 minutes.

6 To finish, inhale deeply and hold your breath. Interlace your fingers with your right thumb on top and bring your palms about 14in (35cm) in front of you at the level of the thymus gland (just below your throat).

7 Pull your fingers forcefully apart as you hold the breath for as long as you can.

8 Exhale when you need to and repeat three more times. Keep up the pressure as you pull your fingers apart – this stimulates the thymus gland, which is directly linked to your immune system.

9 On the last exhalation curl your tongue back in the roof of your mouth and blow the air out through your lips. Relax.

Meditation for Welcoming Love

This meditation opens your heart to self-love and to the love of others. The mantra will cut through any fears or doubts and allow you to access the truth of your heart. It will open you to new possibilities of love and help those people who are searching for more connection with their partner.

I taught this meditation to a woman who was single and fearful of entering into any new relationship, thinking that she would get hurt. After practising this meditation for 40 days she felt more open, inspired and spontaneous. Within a month of finishing it, the person she was really interested in asked her out on a date. She said "yes" and today, three years on, they are still together.

1 Sit in Half Lotus or Easy Pose (see page 86) and close your eyes, focusing at the third eye. Apply a light Neck Lock (see page 72).

2 Bring your hands into Prayer Mudra (see page 121) at the centre of your chest and repeat the mantra SAT KAR TAR ("saat, kaar, taar", meaning "manifestor of the truth") a few times. Roll the "R" each time and keep the flow between the syllables, emphasizing each one evenly.

3 With your hands in Prayer Mudra, say SAT.

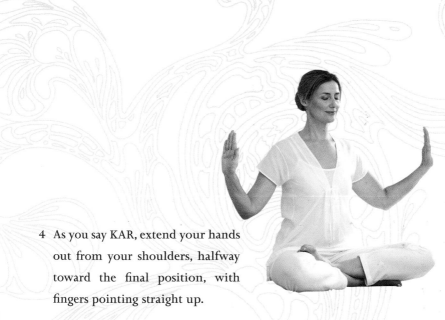

4 As you say KAR, extend your hands out from your shoulders, halfway toward the final position, with fingers pointing straight up.

5 As you say TAR, fully extend your arms out to the sides, parallel to the floor and with your fingers pointing up.

6 Coordinate the movement with the mantra and find your rhythm. Repeat for 3–11 minutes and feel yourself opening and expanding on each repetition of the mantra. Invite love into your life!

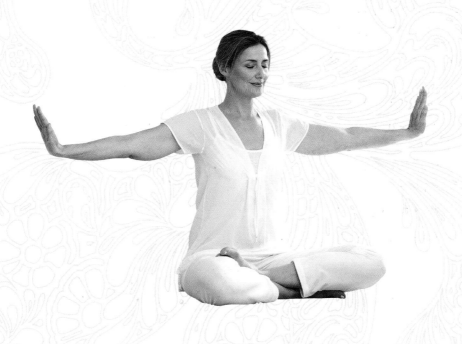

Meditation to Lift Depression

Many people suffer from a mild or acute form of depression at some stage in their lives, including anxiety, unhappiness and identity problems. As a natural alternative to anti-depressants, try practising this meditation daily to help you cope. You will find you have more control over your mind and can cut through the dark cloud of depression to a place of balance, peace and joy.

WAHE GURU is a powerful mantra that takes you from darkness to light, from ignorance to understanding. It invokes Kundalini energy to purify your past karma and to give you vitality. This is the mantra of ecstasy and it will clear away feelings of loneliness, doubt, fear or confusion. I gave this meditation to a student who had sunk into deep depression after losing her mother in a car crash. She said that the mantra was a huge help, lifting her out of a dark place.

1 Sit in Half Lotus or Easy Pose (see page 86) and hold out your hands about 6in (15cm) from your chest in a reversed Prayer Mudra (see page 121). Keep your thumbs separated and your fingers pressed against one another, creating pressure on the back of your hands. Apply a light Neck Lock (see page 72).

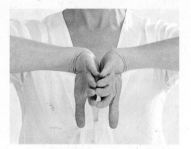

2 Focus your eyes at the tip of your nose.

3 Take a few long, deep breaths in and out of the nostrils to prepare yourself.

4 Inhale deeply and chant WAHE GURU (pronounced "wah-hey goo-roo") 16 times as you breathe out. One complete cycle should take 20–25 seconds.

5 Try this for 11 minutes and gradually build to 31 minutes.

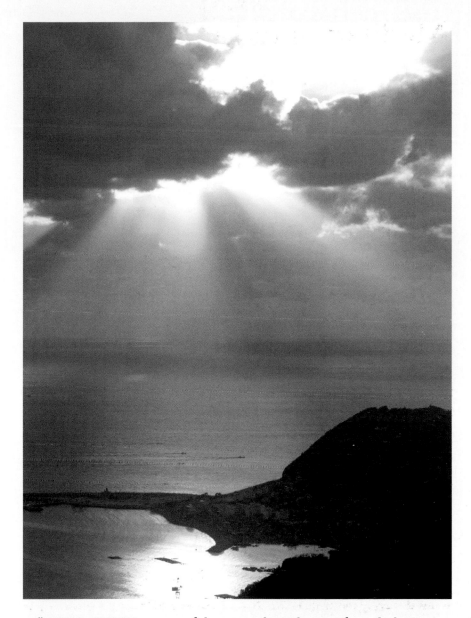

"*WAHE GURU is a powerful mantra that takes you from darkness to light, from ignorance to understanding.*"

Meditation to Awaken Kundalini and Creativity

This meditation, known as Sat Kriya, is great for everyone and can be practised daily. It is very powerful and works on many levels – profound and subtle – of your being. Your internal organs will benefit from the rhythmic pulse at the navel and the flow of your sexual energy will be strengthened. Any imbalances in the lower three chakras will be cleared and sexual phobias will be eased. It is one of the key meditations to awaken Kundalini energy and invite more creativity into your life. Whenever I am feeling blocked creatively and lacking in inspiration, this meditation shifts my energy within a few seconds.

1 Sit in Rock Pose, as pictured opposite. If that is difficult, sit in Easy Pose (see page 86) or on a chair.

2 Interlock your fingers, leaving your index fingers together and extended. Women place the left thumb on top of the right thumb, and men place the right thumb on top of the left thumb.

3 Stretch your arms up high with the index fingers pointing straight up. Try to keep your shoulder blades relaxed as you stretch from the base of the spine to the tips of your index fingers. Apply a light Neck Lock (see page 72).

4 Close your eyes and focus at your third eye. This will stimulate your pituitary gland and awaken your intuition, which is powerfully linked with creativity, and in this meditation you will feel the connection between them.

5 Begin to chant SAT NAM ("sat naam", meaning "truth is my name"), pulling the navel in and up very powerfully on SAT and releasing it on NAM, which is a shorter and softer syllable. Your breath will automatically adjust when you find your rhythm. Continue for 3 minutes.

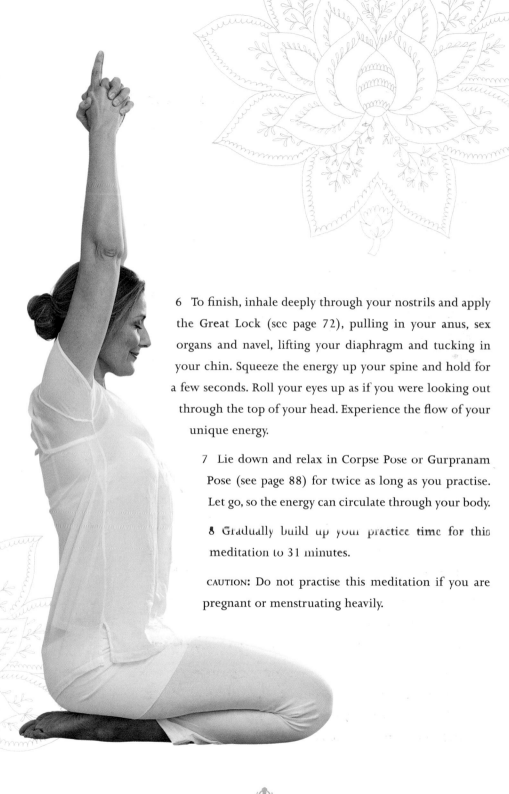

6 To finish, inhale deeply through your nostrils and apply the Great Lock (see page 72), pulling in your anus, sex organs and navel, lifting your diaphragm and tucking in your chin. Squeeze the energy up your spine and hold for a few seconds. Roll your eyes up as if you were looking out through the top of your head. Experience the flow of your unique energy.

7 Lie down and relax in Corpse Pose or Gurpranam Pose (see page 88) for twice as long as you practise. Let go, so the energy can circulate through your body.

8 Gradually build up your practice time for this meditation to 31 minutes.

CAUTION: Do not practise this meditation if you are pregnant or menstruating heavily.

Meditation to Create Abundance

This meditation will guide you through any mental block and give clarity and reassurance about the future. It will activate your neutral, meditative mind, allowing you to intuit expected and unexpected thoughts without anxiety. You will gain wisdom and trust as you open yourself to the flow of prosperity and the abundance of life. I practised this meditation for 40 days in the lead-up to an important audition and got the job, so trust, it does work!

1 Sit in Half Lotus or Easy Pose (see page 86) with a light Neck Lock (see page 72).

2 Close your eyes, focusing attention on your third eye, the invisible point midway between the eyebrows. This will expand your intuition and awareness. Alternatively, you can open your eyes and gently focus them down toward the tip of your nose. This activates the optic nerve, the pineal gland and the frontal lobe of the brain, making your mind calmer and developing your intuition.

3 Relax your elbows down by the sides of your ribcage and bring your forearms parallel to the ground. With your hands pointing forward and your palms facing up, touch your thumbs to the tips of your index fingers.

4 Chant HAR HARAY HAREE WAHE GURU (pronounced "har har-ray ha-ree wah-hey goo-roo"), feeling the ecstasy of the mantra. Visualize yourself opening to health, wealth, happiness, joy and anything you desire.

5 Continue for 3–11 minutes and then sit in silence.

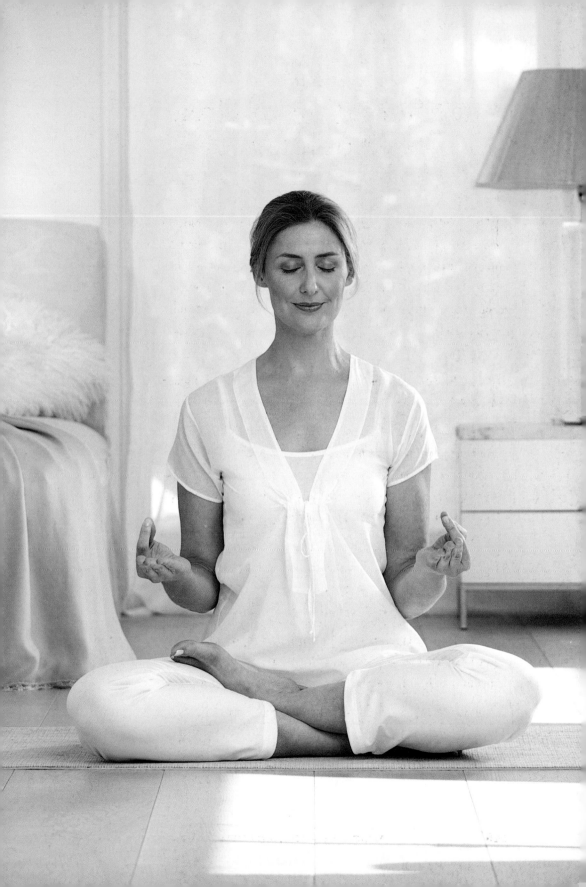

Meditation for a Fresh Start

Known as Sodarshan Chakra Kriya, this is one of the most powerful Kundalini meditations. It will directly stimulate Kundalini energy to release the subconscious negative thoughts that may block you from true fulfilment. If you practise it daily, you will re-establish your personal identity, build your creative energy, increase your intuitive powers and clarify your purpose. You will feel an immense sense of health, happiness and joy in life. This was the first Kundalini meditation I practised and words cannot begin to describe how powerful and transformative it is!

1 Sit in Half Lotus or Easy Pose (see page 86) with a light Neck Lock (see page 72).

2 Keep your eyes open and focus on the tip of your nose. This may make you feel dizzy at first; if so, blink and then carry on. Focusing on the tip of the nose stimulates the optic nerve, pineal gland and frontal lobe of the brain, making you calmer and more intuitive.

3 Relax your left hand on your knee in Gyan Mudra (see page 121).

4 Block your right nostril with your right thumb and inhale slowly and deeply through your left nostril.

5 Suspend your breath and mentally chant WAHE GURU ("wah-hey goo-roo") 16 times. Pump the navel point three times with each repetition: once on WA; once on HE; once on GURU. This makes a total of 48 unbroken navel pumps, which can be challenging. Be patient and take your time.

6 After 16 repetitions, release your right nostril and block your left nostril with your index or little finger. Exhale slowly and deeply through your right nostril.

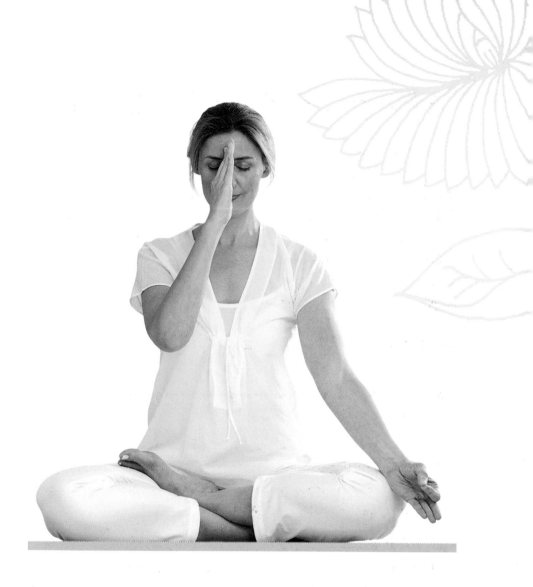

7   Continue repeating Steps 4–6 very slowly for 5 minutes. Gradually build up
    the time to 31 minutes.

8   When you have finished, inhale and suspend your breath for 5–10 seconds.

9   Exhale fully, then stretch your arms up and shake every part of your body for
    a few seconds so that the energy can circulate.

10 Relax in Corpse Pose (see page 88) and feel the transformational effects of
    this powerful meditation!

Meditation for Couples

This meditation allows you the time to really be with your partner. It will remind you of how important it is to take time out to nourish each other's emotional and spiritual needs. Looking into each other's eyes is a powerful technique for opening the heart, and this meditation encourages a deeper connection between you. I often give it to couples who are struggling to listen to and acknowledge one another. The quiet, focused time together is sometimes all it takes to shift the energy in a relationship.

1 Sit in Easy Pose or Half Lotus (see page 86), opposite your partner. Your knees should be almost touching. Adjust your height with a cushion if you cannot comfortably see into your partner's eyes.

2 Each person creates a lotus flower by bringing the base of the hands and the wrists together. All the fingers are spread with only the tips of the little fingers touching.

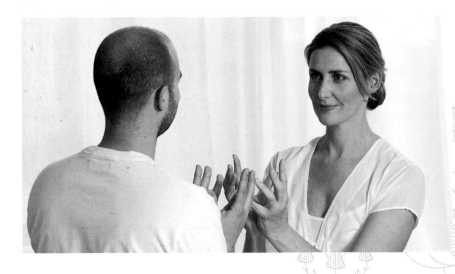

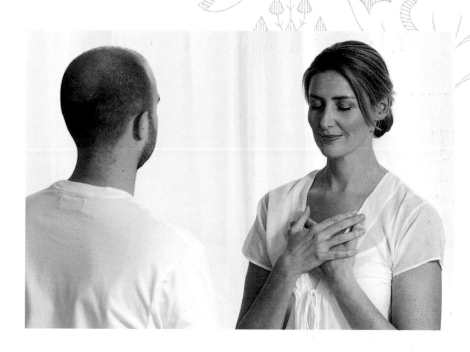

3 The man places his little fingers under the woman's little fingers. These are the only fingers that touch hers, creating a heart lotus. (When this meditation is done with a same-sex partner, decide who takes on the male aspect.)

4 Looking deep into each other's eyes, breathe slowly through your nostrils, synchronizing the rhythm of your breath.

5 Feel the subtle energetic connection as you merge into the divine energy flowing between you. Continue for 1–2 minutes.

6 Now place one hand over another at your heart centre. Close your eyes and meditate on your heart. Go deep within and feel its essence. Be grateful for the time shared with your partner.

7 Continue for 1–2 minutes and then inhale and exhale deeply.

8 Repeat this three times, tuning into your partner's breath.

9 When you have finished, relax to some calming meditative music or show your appreciation by spending time massaging each other.

Meditation for Motherhood

A child's first teacher is his or her mother, and everything begins in the womb. The prayer and protection of a mother is very powerful and this meditation is a beautiful way to have a conversation with your baby when you are pregnant. Be grateful for this precious gift of life and bless your baby.

1 Sit in a comfortable meditation position, stretching tall through your spine. You can use a cushion or a wall to support you if you find it difficult to keep your back straight.

2 Close your eyes and place your left hand on your navel, relaxing your right hand on your knee.

3 Begin long, slow deep breaths through your nostrils, feeling connected to your navel. Let go of any tension as you relax into each breath. Visualize your baby in your womb and consciously communicate with him or her through your calm breath. Do this a few times.

4 Inhale and mentally vibrate SA TA NA MA ("saah, taah, naah, maah") and then exhale, mentally vibrating WAHE GURU ("wah-hey goo-roo"). These sacred words will elevate you and your baby. Feel the sounds as a call to your baby. They will cleanse your solar plexus, heart and throat chakras. Continue for 11 minutes, celebrating the joy of new life.

5 To end, inhale deeply and exhale powerfully three times. Lie down and relax in silence or listen to some soothing music.

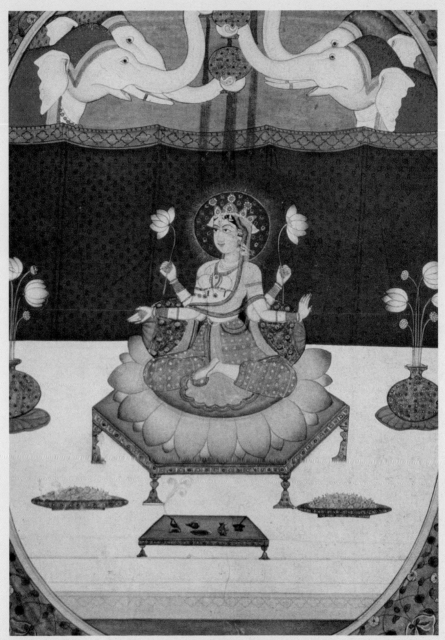

This Indian painting from c. 1660 depicts Lakshmi, wife of Vishnu and goddess of fertility as well of prosperity and beauty, with her lotus symbolizing abundant growth.

MEDITATION FOR MOTHERHOOD

153

Glossary

Adi Mantra primal mantra used to tune in before Kundalini practice

apana outgoing, downward breath; the eliminating energy

asana body position used in yoga

aura field of energy that surrounds and is interconnected to the entire body; the "eighth chakra"

bandha body lock created by pulling internal muscles. The four principal bandhas in Kundalini are Mul Bandh, Uddiyana Bandh, Jalandhara Bandh and Maha Bandh.

bija literally, "seed"; a syllable mantra, such as SAT NAM, that assists in "seeding" consciousness

Buddhi Mudra hand gesture for communication

chakra literally, "circle" or "wheel"; one of seven energy centres of consciousness where the ida and pingala nadis intersect across the sushumna nadi

Golden Chain energetic link to spiritual masters of Kundalini made when chanting the Adi Mantra

Golden Cord energetic connection of crown to third eye chakra made through the pineal, pituitary and hypothalamus glands

guru inner teacher that helps us to move from "dark" to "light" (gu-ru)

Gyan Mudra hand gesture for wisdom, knowledge

higher self soul-consciousness relating to the upper chakras

hydrotherapy yogic science of using cold water with massage to energize the body

ida major nadi, coiling around the sushumna and relating to the left nostril and moon (negative) energy

karma law of cause and effect

kirtan sacred music in which chanting stimulates the pressure points in the upper palate to heighten awareness

kriya posture or sequence of postures linked to a mantra and breathing to produce a particular effect

Kundalini literally, "the coil in the hair of the beloved"; a person's creative potential and divine energy, which lies dormant at the base of the spine and may be activated

Maha Bandha the great lock, created by pulling the three locks – Jalandhara Banda, Mul Bandh and Uddiyana Bandh – at once

mantra rhythmical repetition of a word or syllable that helps to control mental chatter and elevate consciousness

mudra yogic hand gesture

nadi channel of subtle energy within the body

navel point corresponds to the solar plexus chakra; located approximately 2–3in (5–7.5cm) below the umbilicus and the point where the body's 72,000 nadis come together

pingala major nadi, coiling around the sushumna and relating to the right nostril and sun (positive) energy

prana subtle life force; the energy we breathe

pranayama literally "to lead the life force"; the science of yogic breathing exercises

sadhana daily spiritual practice, especially before dawn

samadhi state of consciousness in which the mind is merged within the infinite

Sanskrit earliest-known Indo-European language

SAT NAM literally, "truth identity" or "truth manifested"; seed syllable mantra

Shakti feminine creative principal; creative power of Shiva

Shiva Lord of Yoga, destroyer and creator; represents the male principle

Shuni Mudra hand gesture for patience and self-discipline

Sitali Breath cooling, calming breath

Surya Mudra hand gesture for energy

sushumna central spine channel of chakra system through which Kundalini ascends

Tantra yogic science of applied consciousness, concerning expansion of the subtle energetic body and the psyche

tapa inner psychic "heat" of the prana that comes from repetition of mantras

tattvas five elements of which the universe is composed: fire, air, earth, water and ether

third eye invisible point of focus, midway between the brows, relating to the individual's centre of intuition; also known as the third eye or brow chakra

Vedas four sacred texts composed in India and orally transmitted during *c.* 1500–500/400 BCE; written down, in Sanskrit, after this period

yantra sacred diagram used to balance the mind or focus it on spiritual concepts

yoga literally, "union"; physical and spiritual practices to achieve the union of body, mind and spirit

Further Reading

Avalon, Arthur, *The Serpent Power: The Secrets of Tantric and Shaktic Yoga*, Dover: London, 1974

Bhajan, Yogi, and Khalsa, Gurucharan Singh, *The Mind: Its Projections and Multiple Facets*, Kundalini Research Institute: Santa Cruz, NM, 1998

Bhajan, Yogi, and Khalsa, Shabad Kaur, *The Master's Touch: On Being a Sacred Teacher for the New Age*, Kundalini Research Institute: Santa Cruz, NM, 1997

Judith, Anodea, *Wheels of Life: A User's Guide to the Chakra System*, Llewellyn Worldwide: Woodbury, MN, 1987

Khalsa, Dharma Singh, *Meditation as Medicine: Activate the Power of Your Natural Healing Force*, Simon & Schuster: New York, 2001
—— *Food as Medicine: How to Use Diet, Vitamins, Juices and Herbs for a Healthier, Happier and Longer Life*, Simon and Schuster: New York, 2003

Khalsa, Shakta Kaur, *Kundalini Yoga: Classic Postures and Dynamic Breathing Techniques to Release Energy and Unlock Your Inner Potential*, Dorling Kindersley: London, 2001

Krishnamurti, J., *This Light in Oneself: True Meditation*, Shambhala: Berkeley, CA, 1999

Levry, Joseph Michael, *The Divine Doctor: Healing Beyond Medicine*, Rootlight: Camarillo, CA, 2003

Mookerjee, Ajit, *Kundalini: The Arousal of the Inner Energy*, Thames & Hudson: London, 1982

Newberg, Andrew, and Waldman, Mark R., *How God Changes Your Brain: Breakthrough Findings from a Leading Neuroscientist*, Random House: London, 2009

Osho, *Meditation: The First and Last Freedom*, St Martin's Press: New York, 1996

Saradananda, Swami, *The Power of Breath: The Art of Breathing Well for Harmony, Happiness and Health*, Duncan Baird: London, 2009

Saraswati, Swami Satyananda, *Kundalini Tantra*, Bihar School of Yoga: India, 1984

Shannahoff-Khalsa, David S., *Kundalini Yoga Meditation for Complex Psychiatric Disorders: Techniques Specific for Treating the Psychoses, Personality and Pervasive Development Disorders*, W.W. Norton & Co: London, 2010

Silverton, Sarah, *The Mindfulness Breakthrough*, Watkins Publishing: London, 2012

Tolle, Eckhart, *The Power of Now: A Guide to Spiritual Enlightenment*, Hodder and Stoughton: London, 1999

For more information on the teachings of Yogi Bhajan, visit www.3ho.org or the official website of the Kundalini Research Institute at www.kundaliniresearchinstitute.org

For more on Kathryn McCusker and her work with Kundalini, visit www.kathrynmccuskerkundalini.com

Index

aarti 50
abundance meditation 146
addictions, meditation for 132
Adi-Buddha 30
Adi Mantra 24, 58–9, 119, 154
ajna chakra see third eye chakra
Alternate Nostril Breathing 108
anahata chakra see heart chakra
anger, meditation to release 134
apana vayu 66, 154
   activating 79
   and breath suspension 100
   flow of 94, 68–72
Ardhanarishvara 29
asanas 16, 17, 73–83, 154
awareness, developing 42, 44–5, 48
Ayurveda 56

Baby Pose 87, 88
bandhas 17, 70–2, 94, 154
base chakra 36, 51, 69
   and asanas 16
   and endocrine system 41
   exercises to stimulate 75, 76, 78, 79, 86
   and sounds 119
Bear Grip 123
Bhajan, Yogi 11, 24, 32
bija 118–19, 154
body, purifying the 54–5

body locks 17, 70–2, 94, 154
Brahma 27
brahmani nadi 35
brain, effect of meditation on 14–15
Breath of Fire 107, 110
breathing: breath suspension 94, 97, 100–1
   circular breathing 112–13
   developing breath awareness 98–9
   in Kundalini 17
   into the navel centre 103
   meditations to master breath 106–11
   One-Minute Breath 97
   pranayama 73, 92, 94–7, 120, 155
   and stress 89, 92–3, 98
brow chakra see third eye chakra
Buddha Mudra 122
Buddhi Mudra 121, 130, 154
Buddhism 30, 32, 52, 120, 127

Cannon Breath 110
Cat Pose 80–1
chakras 34, 36–9, 154
   and asanas 16
   and the endocrine system 40–1
   opening with sound 32–3
   using goddesses 51
   yantras 124–7
   see also individual chakras

chitrini nadi 35
Christ Mudra 122
clavicular breathing 98
cleansing meditation 138–9
cleansing ritual 54, 69
clothing for meditation 55
Corpse Pose 88
couples, meditation for 150–1
Cow Pose 80–1
creativity, meditation to awaken 144–5
crown chakra 38, 69
   and the endocrine system 41
   exercises to stimulate 74
   opening 33
   and Prajnaparamita 52

Dalai Lama 30
Davidson, Professor Richard 14–15
depression, and meditation 12, 142
Devi 24, 26–7, 51
   see also Shakti
Diaphragm Lock 69, 70, 71
Durga 27, 52

Easy Pose 16, 33, 86, 120
Ego Eradicator 74
emotions 62–3, 134
   emotional balance meditation 130–1
endocrine system 40–1, 82
energy: awakening 42, 44, 73–83
   and breathing 92

and nadis 68
sexual 29, 112–13
subtle energy system
34–5
see also prana

female and male integration
28–9, 30
food, to aid meditation
56–7
Fredrickson, Dr Barbara 15
fresh start, meditation for
148–9
Frog Pose 16, 79, 80
Full Lotus 16, 120

Gita Govinda 29, 51
goddesses 26–7, 51–2
see also individual incarnations
Golden Chain 24, 154
Great Lock 70, 72
Gurmukhi Mantra 32
Gurpranam Pose 88
Gyan Mudra 121, 130, 154

habits 62–3, 132
Half Lotus 16, 33, 86, 120
healing meditation 136
heart chakra 29, 37
and the endocrine system
41
exercises to stimulate 74
opening 33
and Parvati 52
Hinduism 27, 28, 32, 120,
127
hydrotherapy 54, 154

ida nadi 35, 68, 94, 154
immune system, boosting
138–9

inspiration, finding 49
integration 28
intuition meditation 130–1

Jalandhara Bandha 70, 72
Janaka of Mithila, King 24
Jung, Carl 42

Kabat-Zinn, Jon 15
Kali 27
Kirtan Kriya meditation 15,
130–1
Krishna 29, 51
Krishna, Gopi 42
kriya 154
Kundalini: definition 22–3,
154
flow of 68–9
meditation to awaken
144–5
origins 24
in other traditions 30
power of 12–13
and your well-being
14–15

Lakshmi 27
letting go 63, 89
Lion Breath 111
listening, deep 60
Live Nerve Stretch 78
long, deep breathing 106–7
Lotus Mudra 123
love, meditation for
welcoming 140–1
loving-kindness meditation
15

Maha Bandha 70, 72, 154
Mahisa 27, 52
male and female integration

28–9, 30
manipura chakra *see* solar
plexus chakra
mantras 17, 32, 116–19,
154
and activating nadis 68
and opening chakras 33
and tuning in 58–9
mindfulness meditation 15
motherhood meditation 152
mudras 17, 54, 120–3, 155
and mantras 130
and opening chakras 33
Mul Bandha 70
muladhara chakra *see* base
chakra

nadis 34–5, 155
and flow of Kundalini
68, 94
and the navel centre 83,
103
navel centre 83, 102–5, 107,
155
Neck Lock 69, 70, 72, 120
Neck Rolls 16, 82–3
negativity 62–3, 84, 138
Nostril Breathing, Alternate
108
nyasa 54

One-Minute Breath 97

Parvati 27, 29, 52
pineal gland 22, 41, 132
pingala nadi 35, 68, 94, 155
poses for meditation 84–9
Prajnaparamita 52
prana 66–9, 155
and breath suspension
100

and breathing 92
building awareness 104–5
effect of negativity on 84
flow of 94, 106, 120
and food 56
see also energy
prana vayu 67, 68–72
pranayama 73, 92, 94–7, 120, 155
Prayer Mudra 121
Praying Mantis Mudra 122
pregnancy meditation 152
purifying the body 54–5, 69

Radha 29, 51
rajasic foods 57
Ram Das, Guru 24
relaxation poses 84–9
Rock Pose 87, 120
root chakra *see* base chakra
Root Lock 69, 70

sacral chakra 37
   and the endocrine system 41
   exercises to stimulate 76, 79, 80
   opening 33
   and Radha 51
sadhana 54, 155
sahasrara chakra *see* crown chakra
samadhi 155
samana vayu 66
Sanskrit 116, 118, 119, 155
Sarasvati 27, 52
Sat Kriya 144–5
sattvic foods 56–7
Seed Mantra 119
seed syllables 118–19
sexual energy: and circular

breathing 112–13
and Kundalini 29
Shakti 22, 26–9, 32, 127, 155
Shava-asana 88
Shiva 22, 28–9, 118, 155
   and Parvati 52
   Sri Yantra 127
   and the Tantras 24
shrines 50
Shuni Mudra 121, 130, 155
Sikhism 120
Singh, Karta 11
Siri Gaitri Mantra 136
Sitali Breath 111, 155
Sodarshan Chakra Kriya 63, 148–9
solar plexus chakra 37, 69, 94
   and Durga 52
   and the endocrine system 41
   exercises to stimulate 74, 76, 79, 80
   the navel centre 102–5
   opening 33
sound 32–3, 116–19
   see also mantras
spaces for meditation 50–3
Spinal Flexes 75
Sri Yantra (Sri Chakra) 127
stress 12, 89, 92–3, 98
Stretch Pose 83, 104–5
subtle energy system 34–5
Sufi Grinds 76
Sukasana 86
Surya Mudra 121, 130, 155
sushumna nadi 35, 68, 69, 155
svadhisthana chakra *see* sacral chakra

Tantrism 24, 30, 124
   circular breathing 112
   and the Great Goddess 26–7
   and integration 17, 28
   Tantras 24, 94, 155
   tantrikas 54
Tara 52
tension, letting go of 89
third eye chakra 38, 69, 155
   and the endocrine system 41
   exercises to stimulate 74
   opening 33
   and Tara 52
throat chakra 38, 69
   and the endocrine system 41
   opening 33, 111
   and Sarasvati 52
   tuning in 58–9

udana vayu 67
Uddiyana Bandha 70, 71
University of California (UCLA) 15

vajra nadi 30, 35
Vajrayana Buddhism 30, 87
Vedas 28, 155
Venus Lock 17, 122
Vishnu 24, 27
visualization 99
vishuddha chakra *see* throat chakra
vyana vayu 67

Whistle Breath 110

yantras 24, 124–7, 155
Yoni Mudra 17, 123

Acknowledgments

Author acknowledgments

I have encountered many wonderful people on my travels and through my passion for music and yoga. All of them have either inspired and supported me in my professional life or have somehow influenced and shaped my growth and awareness. I would like to take this opportunity to thank them all for contributing to my life and so enriching the vision for this book.

Special thanks go to: my publisher Duncan Baird for having the confidence in me to explore a book about Kundalini meditation; my editors, Sandra Rigby and Fiona Robertson, for their unswerving patience and understanding throughout the process; my teachers, especially Karta Singh, who awakened my curiosity and opened my eyes to a fresh and creative way of interpreting Kundalini; and my students and colleagues for their trust and support, in particular those whose stories have been included in this book.

Finally, love and gratitude go to my husband Paul for his unconditional support and understanding from the beginning to the end.

SAT NAM

Picture acknowledgments

The publisher would like to thank the following people, museums and photographic libraries for permission to reproduce their material. Every care has been taken to trace copyright holders. However, if we have omitted anyone we apologize and will, if informed, make corrections to any future edition.

Page 19 Gerolf Kalt/Corbis; **23** R. u. S. Michaud/akg-images; **25** © Victoria and Albert Museum, London; **28** Hal Beral/Visuals Unlimited/Corbis; **31** Thierry Ollivier/Musée Guimet, Paris/(C) RMN; **36–8** Dreamstime; **39** British Library/The Art Archive; **45** R. u. S. Michaud/akg-images; **50** Radius Images/Alamy; **53** Monique Pietri/akg-images; **57** Dr. Neil Overy/Stockfood; **61** Vaclav Volrab/Shutterstock; **71** Dreamstime; **77** Chris Knorr/Design Pics/Corbis; **85** © The Trustees of the British Museum; **96** R. u. S. Michaud/akg-images; **102** Hany Maurice Photo/Getty Images; **109** Philippe Sainte-Laudy Photography/Getty Images; **117** Ian Cumming/Axiom; **118** Museum of Fine Arts, Houston, Texas/Gift of Carol & Robert Straus/The Bridgeman Art Library; **125** Dreamstime; **126** Science Museum/Science & Society Picture Library/Getty Images; **133** Arthur Morris/Getty Images; **143** Yuji Higashida/Getty Images; **153** Private Collection/Ann & Bury Peerless Picture Library/The Bridgeman Art Library.